Recent Titles in
Contributions in Afro-American and African Studies

African American Autobiography and the Quest for Freedom
Roland L. Williams, Jr.

The White Image in the Black Mind: A Study of African American Literature
Jane Davis

Black Leadership for Social Change
Jacob U. Gordon

Mythatypes: Signatures and Signs of African/Diaspora and Black Goddesses
Alexis Brooks De Vita

African Visions: Literary Images, Political Change, and Social Struggle in Contemporary Africa
Cheryl B. Mwaria, Silvia Federici, and Joseph McLaren, editors

Voices of the Fugitives: Runaway Slave Stories and Their Fictions of Self-Creation
Sterling Lecater Bland, Jr.

Meditations on African Literature
Dubem Okafor

Achebe the Orator: The Art of Persuasion in Chinua Achebe's Novels
Chinwe Christiana Okechukwu

Rethinking the Slave Narrative: Slave Marriage and the Narratives of Henry Bibb and William and Ellen Craft
Charles J. Heglar

The Harlem Group of Negro Writers
Melvin B. Tolson
Edward J. Mullen, editor

Rereading the Harlem Renaissance: Race, Class, and Gender in the Fiction of Jessie Fauset, Zora Neale Hurston, and Dorothy West
Sharon L. Jones

Critical Essays on Bessie Head
Maxine Sample, editor

REPRODUCTION AND SOCIAL CONTEXT IN SUB-SAHARAN AFRICA

A Collection of Micro-Demographic Studies

Edited by Samuel Agyei-Mensah and John B. Castberline
Foreword by George Benneh

Contributions in Afro-American and African Studies, Number 206

GREENWOOD PRESS
Westport, Connecticut • London

Library of Congress Cataloging-in-Publication Data

Reproduction and social context in sub-Saharan Africa : a collection of micro-demographic studies / edited by Samuel Agyei-Mensah and John B. Casterline ; foreword by George Benneh.
p. cm. — (Contributions in Afro-American and African studies, ISSN 0069-9624 ; no. 206)
Includes bibliographical references and index.
ISBN 0-313-31908-1 (alk. paper)
1. Fertility, Human—Africa, Sub-Saharan. 2. Birth control—Africa, Sub-Saharan. I. Agyei-Mensah, Samuel, 1961- II. Casterline, J. B. III. Series.
HB1071.A3 R467 2003
304.6'32'0967—dc21 2002024483

British Library Cataloguing in Publication Data is available.

Library of Congress Catalog Card Number: 2002024483
ISBN: 0-313-31908-1
ISSN: 0069-9624

First published in 2003

Greenwood Press, 88 Post Road West, Westport, CT 06881
An imprint of Greenwood Publishing Group, Inc.
www.greenwood.com

The paper used in this book complies with the Permanent Paper Standard issued by the National Information Standards Organization (Z39.48-1984).

10 9 8 7 6 5 4 3 2 1

Contents

Foreword

It is a privilege to be asked to preface this interesting collection of chapters. Coming from a background in geography with a specialty in environmental and population issues, I have been fascinated with the tremendous diversity in environmental and population issues between and within the societies of sub-Saharan Africa. It is this idea of place and geographic uniqueness that I find most interesting and revealing of the chapters presented in this volume.

The chapters adhere essentially to microdemography. Clearly the editors have made an effort to extend beyond the traditional notions of microdemography articulated by John Caldwell some decades ago, with its emphasis on anthropological and ethnographic studies, to a more inclusive approach. Central to the editors' understanding of microdemography is the emphasis on localized contextual studies, and the use of both qualitative and quantitative methodologies. Indeed, it is the localized character of these studies that permits investigators to probe certain topics more intensively than is feasible in studies with broader geographic coverage, such as studies relying on the World Fertility Surveys and Demographic and Health Surveys. Perhaps most important, when studies are localized, investigators are almost compelled to be more sensitive to local context.

I feel that the original aim of the editors has been achieved: the chapters in this volume effectively demonstrate how microdemographic research can extend our knowledge of reproductive behavior and reproductive change in sub-Saharan Africa beyond what can be learned from national aggregate studies. Consistent with the editors' view that the microdemographic approach should not be equated with qualitative research, the volume contains a mix of quantitative and qualitative methodologies, although on balance quantitative research is the more dominant in this set of studies. It is my hope that this volume makes a persuasive case for the value of rigorous quantitative microdemographic research.

The geographic coverage is most impressive, spanning seven countries. A diverse set of topics is discussed, ranging from adolescent fertility and reproductive decision making, to social identity and minority group influences on fertility, to the impact of development programs, social organization, and birth timing on fertility change. I note with much satisfaction the diversity of disciplines represented, which include demography, geography, sociology, public health, anthropology, and economics. The authors are both African and non-African, and among Africans are from Sahelian, West, East, and Southern Africa, representing both anglophone and francophone countries.

The volume is a timely contribution to fresh thinking and theorizing on demographic concepts and knowledge on the African fertility transition. It will be a great resource for population experts, students, and policymakers.

George Benneh

Acknowledgments

We began our work on this volume in 1999 with some anxiety about the prospects for success, given the objectives we had set for ourselves. The very nature of microdemography invited skepticism. Our initial fears were allayed with the acceptance of the proposal by Greenwood Press. Since then, we have shepherded the project through each phase, motivated by our shared commitment to extend beyond the traditional boundaries of microdemography and by our belief that geography and locality ought to be recognized in demographic enquiry, especially in sub-Saharan Africa.

The assembling and editing of the volume took place in both Ghana and the United States, through occasional meetings in both countries and innumerable e-mail exchanges in between. At various turns, we faced difficult choices. Throughout, we have attempted to maintain high intellectual standards and an allegiance to the main objectives motivating the volume. We thank the authors for their willingness to adhere to deadlines and for their responsiveness to the editors' requests for revisions. More often than not, these requests included deletion of substantial portions of manuscripts, in order to keep the volume within the overall length limits, and naturally this was painful for authors. We take this opportunity to express our thanks to all the contributors, especially John and Pat Caldwell for the concluding chapter.

We also appreciate the wonderful work by everyone at Greenwood Press involved with the project, especially the acquisitions editor, Cynthia Harris, and our production editor, Megan Peckman. Finally, we thank Doreen Totaram of the Population Council, New York for preparing the camera-ready pages.

1

REPRODUCTION AND SOCIAL CONTEXT IN SUB-SAHARAN AFRICA: AN INTRODUCTION

Samuel Agyei-Mensah and John B. Casterline

During the past three decades, demographic research in sub-Saharan Africa has made substantial strides forward. With the availability of demographic survey data from the World Fertility Surveys (WFS) in the late 1970s and early 1980s and the Demographic and Health Surveys (DHS) from the mid-1980s to the present, there has been an acceleration in both the quantity and quality of research. It is now relatively easy to analyze demographic data from many African countries, and to carry out sophisticated analyses of fertility patterns and their determinants.

Despite the significant contributions of these standardized survey programs, for the purpose of developing in-depth understanding of reproductive regimes in sub-Saharan Africa they suffer from serious limitations. By design these surveys provide a national perspective. Tabulations by region and socio-economic group are generally incidental to the overarching purpose of estimating national parameters. Alternatively, research with these data is from the perspective of the individual; this is the frame of reference of the many published papers that use regression analysis to examine the covariates of reproductive behavior, child survival, and related variables. Only a few scholars, with considerable creativity and determination, have broken from this pattern and analyzed the national survey data from a perspective other than the nation or the individual (see, for example, Tabutin and Schoumaker 2001). Fundamental features of the design of these surveys (their sample design, the content of their questionnaires) preclude careful study of local context—"situating fertility," in Greenhalgh's memorable phrase (Greenhalgh 1995). This insensitivity to microlevel patterns and variations is an especially grave loss in sub-Saharan Africa, home to a very large number of ethnic groups, each with distinctive kinship systems and norms about reproductive behavior. Moreover, the dominance of the major religions is markedly less than in other regions, and national governments are relatively weak. This is not an indictment of the national surveys—without question they serve an indispensable purpose—rather a call for more localized studies that complement the national surveys (Ware 1994). Such localized studies of demographic behavior and its determinants can be collected under the label "microdemographic studies" (Caldwell et al. 1988a).

Our vision of a microdemographic enterprise is not one built entirely on anthropological evidence. Neither do we equate it solely with nonnumerical data. The dominance of anthropological microdemographic studies has led to an erroneous impression that microdemographic studies are optimally anthropological, with quantitative materials entirely absent or at least inessential. (One might get this impression from those volumes that popularized the term; see, for instance, Caldwell et al. 1988a; Caldwell et al. 1988b.) This is an unnecessary restriction. A microdemographic enterprise is first and foremost local and based on small-scale studies. With this as a central characteristic, different research methodologies can be applied, in various combinations. The chapters in this volume are meant to achieve the objective of blending both numerical and nonnumerical data. In this respect, this volume departs from the first generation of microdemography, with its preference for qualitative (and even ethnographic) methodologies and long-term residence in communities.

One of our aims was to assemble a volume that is revealing of the great diversity in Africa, and hence we have tried to include studies from as many different subregions of the continent as possible. The volume contains studies from Sahelian West Africa (Mali), coastal western Africa (Ghana), the horn of Africa (Sudan and Ethiopia), eastern Africa (Kenya and Malawi), and southern African (Zambia). The only major subregion entirely neglected in this volume is central Africa. Concurrently, we have deliberately tried to represent different stages of the African fertility transition: fertility decline is well underway in the study sites in Ghana, Kenya, and Zambia (total fertility rates [TFR] below five births per woman), whereas little decline had occurred at the time of the data collection in Mali, Sudan, Ethiopia, and Malawi (total fertility rates probably in excess of six births per woman).

During the past decade, several volumes and special issues of journals have focused on the fertility transition in sub-Saharan Africa (Foote et al. 1993; Locoh and Hertrich 1994; *Journal of Biosocial Science* 1994; *Journal of International Development* 1995). A number of widely read articles have also examined this topic (van de Walle and Foster 1990; Caldwell et al. 1992; Thomas and Muvandi 1994; Cohen 1998; Kirk and Pillet 1998). With the exception of Caldwell et al. (1992), however, none of these have drawn primarily on microdemographic studies. And previous edited volumes on microdemographic research were far broader in their coverage than this volume, including chapters from Africa and Asia and encompassing not only fertility but also migration and mortality (see Caldwell et al. 1988a). The present volume is far more focused and restricted to contemporary fertility and reproductive health issues in sub-Saharan Africa.

The volume does not pretend to be comprehensive. Many important issues are barely touched on or entirely ignored. For example, none of the chapters deal with current topical issues such as the role of environmental degradation/ agricultural adversity on fertility (see Adjamagbo and Delaunay 1998). And, as already noted, none of the studies was conducted in central Africa. Nevertheless, the volume does bring together new perspectives and original research that was designed to address specific topics. Herein lies an important difference between edited volumes with a central theme and this volume that contains studies of diverse topics, all of them situated within a specific and well-defined context.

The chapters are all original contributions solicited by the editors. The volume consists of ten chapters, including this introduction and a concluding chapter. Following the introduction, Agyeman and Casterline present analysis of data collected in Ghana since 1998. The chapter draws on two research traditions—social organization and social diffusion—in an effort to explain variations in reproductive behavior among six communities along the southern coast of Ghana. The general conclusion is that an explanatory framework that places social organization on center stage must be enlarged to incorporate the potentially powerful influence of community history.

Chapter 3, by Hogan and Berhanu, considers a closely related set of questions about the association between social identity and fertility in southern Ethiopia. One key empirical finding is that minority status has no consistent impact on marriage and reproductive outcomes. Women who live in heterogenous communities do not differ from women in more homogeneous communities in average reproductive outcomes, but they do show more variation in those outcomes.

Chapter 4, by Osman, examines the impact on fertility of a development project, the Rayad Irrigation Project in northern Sudan. Osman discovers that, contrary to prevalent expectations about the association between development projects and fertility, participation in the development project *increases* fertility. Among the explanations he proposes for this surprising finding are the relative availability of health services in the project area, the low cost of raising children, and the absence of family planning services.

Chapter 5, by Agyei-Mensah, Aase, and Awusabo-Asare, a study set in roughly the same geographic area as Agyeman and Casterline, examines the relationship between birth timing and subsequent fertility in three distinct types of locales: affluent urban neighborhoods, poor urban neighborhoods, and poor rural communities. The study reveals that among the urban poor in the capital city of Accra, early childbearing does not necessarily lead to subsequent high fertility. In general, the urban elite delay the onset of childbearing, which translates into subsequent low fertility, whereas the rural poor begin childbearing early and end up with relatively large families. The explanations are sought within the framework of individual/family characteristics, societal change, and ideational influences.

Chapter 6, by Zulu and Kalipeni, examines the linkages between gender relations and the exercise of reproductive control in Malawi. Their results are striking and provocative: while men have played a passive role in decision making concerning traditional methods of child spacing, leaving women considerable reproductive freedom in the past, they now demand to be more directly involved and consulted before their wives adopt modern contraceptives. The chapter contains a rich portrait of the transition underway from more traditional to more modern modes of fertility control.

Chapter 7, by Biddlecom and Kaona, examines factors underlying unmet need for contraception in the small city of Ndola, in the Copperbelt province of Zambia. They observe that contraceptive users and those with unmet need hardly differ with respect to the various hypothesized obstacles to contraceptive use that they consider, such as the strength of attachment to fertility preferences and the social approval of contraception. In common with the Zulu and Kalipeni study in neighboring Malawi, Biddlecom and Kaona provide an in-depth and insightful look at contraceptive logic in a setting where there is substantial demand for control of reproduction but aversion to modern contraceptive technology.

Chapter 8, by Nii-Amoo Dodoo, Sloan, and Zulu, is situated in the slums of Nairobi. The authors examine the confluence of space, context, and hardship on sexual activity among children aged between 13 and 17. The main thesis is that the social, physical, and economic conditions of Kenyan slums combine to normalize early sexual behavior. The analysis draws primarily on highly revealing qualitative interviews.

Adolescent sexuality is also the focus of Chapter 9, by Castle and Konate. They explore the economic context of sexual relations among unmarried sexually active adolescents in rural and urban Mali. Their findings indicate not only that the direction of economic transfers goes from boys to girls, but also that the majority of unmarried girls have, at some point, given gifts or cash to their sexual partner after sexual relations.

In the concluding chapter, John C. Caldwell and Pat Caldwell begin with an overview of the global fertility transition, situating reproductive stability and change in sub-Saharan African during the past two decades in that larger context. Fertility decline has reached Africa last of the major regions of the world, and indeed a majority of the countries in the region have as yet shown little, if any, decline. The Caldwells place the empirical evidence from the set of microdemographic studies assembled in this volume against this backdrop. They use the findings from these studies to draw inferences about future prospects.

REFERENCES

Adjamagbo, A., and V. Delaunay. (1998). The Crisis in the rural West African environment: social implications and effect on fertility. Niakhar (Senegal) and Sassandra (Cote d'Ivoire) compared. *Universites Francophones Actulite Scientifique.*

Caldwell, J.C., A.G. Hill, and V.J. Hull. (1988a). *Micro-Approaches to Demographic Research.* New York: Kegan Paul International.

Caldwell, J.C., P.H. Reddy, and P. Caldwell. (1988b). *The Causes of Demographic Change. Experimental Research in South India.* Madison: University of Wisconsin Press.

Caldwell, J.C., I. Oruboloye, and P. Caldwell (1992). Fertility decline in Africa: A new type of transition. *Population and Development Review* 19(2): 211–242.

Cohen, B. (1998). The emerging fertility transition in sub-Saharan Africa. *World Development*. 26(8): 1431–1461.

Foote, K., K. Hill, and L. Martin (eds). (1993). *Demographic Change in Sub-Saharan Africa*. Washington, D.C.: National Academy Press.

Greenhalgh, S. (1995). *Situating Fertility. Anthropology and Demographic Enquiry*. Cambridge: Cambridge University Press.

Journal of Biosocial Science. (1994). Special Issue on fertility transition in sub-Saharan Africa.

Journal of International Development. (1995). Special Issue on fertility transition in Sub-Saharan Africa.

Kirk, D., and B. Pillet. (1998). Fertility levels, trends, and determinants in sub-Saharan Africa in the 1980s and 1990s. *Studies in Family Planning* 29(1): 1–22.

Locoh, T. and V. Hertrich. (eds.). (1994). *The Onset of Fertility Transition in sub-Saharan Africa*. Liege, Belgium: Ordina Editions.

Tabutin, D., and B. Schoumaker. (2001). Une analyse régionale des transitions de fécondité en Afrique sub-saharienne. Paper presented at IUSSP General Conference, Salvador, Brazil, August 18–24, 2001.

Thomas, D., and I. Muvandi. (1994). The demographic transition in Southern Africa: reviewing the evidence from Botswana and Zimbabwe. *Demography* 31(2): 217–227.

Van de Walle, E., and A. Foster. (1990). *Fertility Decline in Africa: assessment and prospects*. World Bank Technical Paper no. 125, Africa Technical Department Series. Washington, D.C.: World Bank.

Ware, H. (1994). Thoughts on the course of fertility transition in sub-Saharan Africa. Pp. 289–296 in T. Locoh and V. Hetrich (eds.). *The Onset of Fertility Transition in sub-Saharan Africa*. Liege, Belgium: Ordina Editions.

2

SOCIAL ORGANIZATION AND REPRODUCTIVE BEHAVIOR IN SOUTHERN GHANA

Dominic K. Agyeman and John B. Casterline

INTRODUCTION

This chapter joins together two research traditions that have attempted to explain societal-level variation in fertility. Both traditions have long heritages and large literatures. The first tradition posits that reproductive behavior is heavily influenced by the social organization and cultural practices of a society. While this proposition can be applied to any society, whatever its cultural heritage or level of income (or, for that matter, level of fertility), perhaps in no region has this proposition held greater sway over research on reproduction than in sub-Saharan Africa, going back at least to the seminal volume edited by Lorimer in the 1950s (Lorimer 1954), continuing with much originality in Caldwell's papers in the late 1970s (Caldwell 1982), and revived once more in the stimulating set of papers collected by Lesthaeghe in his 1989 volume (Lesthaeghe 1989) and the ambitious multivolume National Academy of Sciences assessment of the demography of sub-Saharan Africa (NRC 1993). The proposition can be broken into several distinct subpropositions—social organization can be distinguished from cultural practices, and both subdivided further—but a common mode of analysis unites the various strands in this research tradition: societal-level variation in reproduction is explained by the imperatives contained in the cultural and social systems that have been passed down across the generations. The key imperatives might concern childbearing itself, or any one of the chief proximate determinants of fertility, such as marriage and the postpartum behaviors. This school of thought struggles to explain reproductive change. This is not to say that the major theoretical frameworks linking social organization and reproductive behavior cannot comfortably accommodate reproductive change, but one must look outside this research tradition for a full-fledged theory for why, and how, reproductive change might occur.

Social change is the main preoccupation of the second research tradition that informs the work in this chapter. The innovation diffusion tradition posits that social change can occur as the result of novel ideas, technologies, and behaviors spreading from one social group to another (Rogers 1983). Obviously individuals must perceive that adoption of the innovation will be to their advantage, but cost-benefit analysis that favors the innovation is not in itself sufficient: individuals must be exposed to the innovative ideas, technologies, and behaviors, and ordinarily this requires their introduction from the outside, i.e., innovation diffusion. There are several means by which innovations can be introduced into a group. This might occur deliberately through the mass media or formal schooling, as has been the case with modern contraception in sub-Saharan Africa (and other high-fertility societies) in recent decades. Perhaps more interesting from a social scientific standpoint, and more challenging as well, is innovation diffusion through social networks. This channel is comprised of various mechanisms, including informal day-to-day conversation with friends and neighbors, discussion with workmates, and exchanges in formal group meetings. Social networks vary in size and structure from one society to another, and this may well have implications for the ease and rapidity of innovation diffusion (Valente 1995). A common argument, to which we return below, makes a distinction between homogeneous and heterogeneous networks, with the latter on balance facilitating innovation diffusion. Henceforth in this chapter, the phrase "social diffusion" will be used to refer to innovation diffusion that occurs through social networks, broadly defined.

It is the linkage between social organization and social diffusion, in this instance with respect to reproductive behavior, that is the primary interest in this chapter. The aim is not to put the validity of either research tradition to a fundamental test, rather by joining them to gain insights about how social organization can affect reproductive behavior. The analytical strategy for achieving this end is comparison of a discrete number of communities in southern Ghana, first characterizing their social organization, then considering how the communities vary in their receptivity to social diffusion, and finally examining covariation of both with indicators of reproductive behavior (fertility and its proximate determinants). Because fertility is declining in Ghana, with increased practice of modern contraception a major contributing factor (Ghana Statistical Service and Macro International 1999; Blanc and Grey 2000), there is good reason to posit that the receptivity of these communities to innovative reproductive behavior (itself in part a function of social organizational features) will explain much of the observed cross-community variation in reproductive behavior. In linking social organization to social diffusion, we depart from the concerns of Caldwell (1982) and Lesthaeghe (1989), who consider social organizations in relation to modes of production and reproduction, which leads to a theoretical framework for reproductive behavior that contains a heavy emphasis on economic arguments. In contrast, the present chapter focuses on the role of social organizations and other social structures as mechanisms/channels of social diffusion.

It should be clear from the preceding paragraphs that this chapter takes the view that reproductive behavior is socially determined and not simply an attribute of an individual. Both research traditions—social organization and innovation diffusion—make this assumption, whether or not explicitly stated. This means that group membership can have considerable bearing on individuals' fertility decisions. As sociologists, this places this chapter squarely in a theoretical tradition that is most prominently represented by Durkheim, and to only a slightly lesser extent by Marx. In keeping with the aim of explaining group-level variation, the analysis in this chapter is carried out at the community level.

DATA

This chapter analyzes data collected in six communities in southern Ghana: two in the Greater Accra Region (Amanfro and Tubaman), two in the Central Region (Brenu-Akyinim and Frami), and two in the Western region (Abuesi and Komfoeku) (see Figure 2.1). The six communities were purposely selected for diversity in ecological setting (coastal versus inland), primary economic activity (farming, fishing, trading), ethnic composition (Ga-Adangbe and Akan) and corresponding kinship (patrilineal and matrilineal), and religion (Christian, Muslim, indigenous). These differences are explored in greater detail in the remainder of this chapter.

Data collection in these sites began in 1994 and has continued up to the present. The analysis in this chapter draws on three types of empirical materials gathered in the six communities:

Community descriptions [henceforth *Community Portrait*]. In 1994/95, and again in 1998/99, project investigators developed relatively in-depth portraits of the study communities, on the basis of extended stays in each community during which formal and informal interviews were conducted and activity in the community was observed. The Community Portraits focus on the political organization of the community, principal economic activities and sources of income, social and religious organizations, schools and health services, and fertility-related customs and practices. While these community descriptions are not proper full-length ethnographic studies, in a more modest fashion they achieve the aim of describing key social organizational features of each community.

Inventory of organizations [henceforth *Organization Inventory*]. In 2000, an inventory of organizations in each community was constructed, through interviews with members of each community. The intention was to obtain a comprehensive listing of organizations in each community—the name of the organization, its objectives, number of members, and frequency of meeting.

Longitudinal survey [henceforth *Panel Survey*]. Women of reproductive age (ages 18–50) and their male partners in each community were first interviewed at length in late 1998, and subsequently have been reinterviewed at roughly six-month intervals in a "panel survey" design. (This chapter makes use of data from rounds 1–3.) The survey sample size for the six communities combined is approximately 1,300 women and 700 male partners. Among the topics inquired about in the Panel Survey are: reproductive behavior (including detailed inquiry about the respondent's reproductive career and his/her contraceptive attitudes and practices); attitudes and preferences concerning childbearing and childrearing; socioeconomic characteristics of the respondent and his/her

Fig. 2.1
Southern Ghana Showing the Study Communities

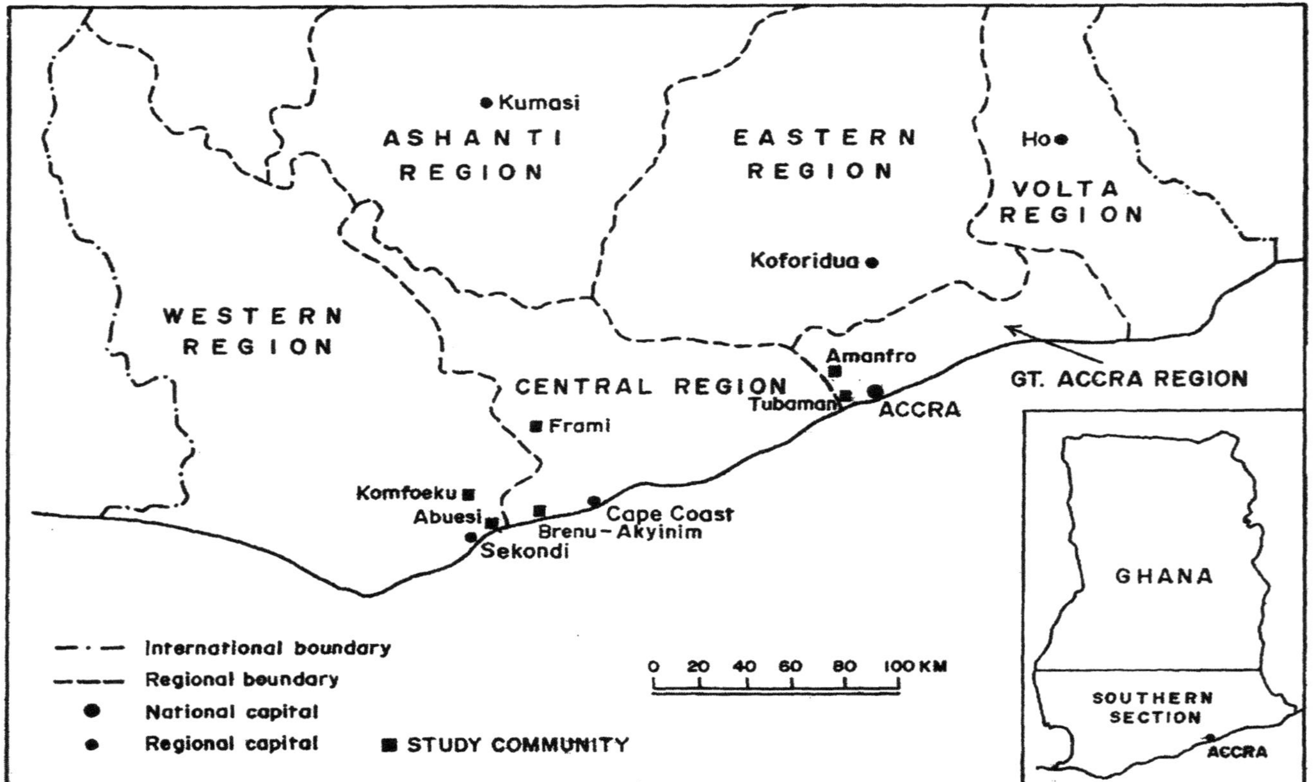

household; knowledge and attitudes about HIV/AIDS; mass media exposure; geographic mobility; social networks.

THE COMMUNITIES

As noted above, the analytical approach in this chapter consists of three stages: a characterization of key social organizational features of each community; a consideration of how these features in turn bear on the receptivity of the communities to social diffusion; and an examination of differentials across communities in reproductive behavior, in light of community differences in social organization and social diffusion receptivity.

BASIC FEATURES

As a means of becoming acquainted with the six communities, their basic features are summarized in Table 2.1. In terms of ecological setting, four of the communities are inland and two coastal. Fishing is a primary economic activity in the two coastal communities, although in fact farming figures as importantly, or more importantly, in the local economy of Brenu-Akyinim. Judging by the mean number of household possessions (items such as radio, television, refrigerator, bed with foam mattress, bicycle, and so forth—ten items maximum) and the percentage of households that are electrified, Amanfro and Tubaman are the more prosperous communities (probably due to their proximity to Accra), and Brenu-Akyinim, Frami, and Komfoeku the less prosperous. The educational attainment of women is highest in Brenu-Akyinim and lower in Abuesi, Komfoeku, and Tubaman, whereas the educational attainment of men is higher in Amanfro and Frami and lower in Abuesi and Tubaman.

There are very interesting differences among the six communities in their religious composition. Tubaman is almost entirely Muslim, and there is a substantial Muslim minority in Abuesi (about one-quarter of respondents). The progression of Islam into West Africa for the most part stopped short of the coast (Islam, of course, is the dominant religion in many parts of the interior of West Africa), but there are nevertheless some significant Muslim communities along the coast. Among the other four communities, affiliation with orthodox Christian denominations predominates in Brenu-Akyinim, whereas Pentecostal Christianity predominates in Amanfro. Frami and Komfoeku are roughly evenly divided between the orthodox and Pentecostal Christians. All the communities, with the exception of Tubaman, permit indigenous religious practices in addition to Christianity and Islam.

Finally, ethnolinguistically four of the communities are comprised primarily of Akan-speaking people (Denkyira in Frami, Fante in the other three), one is predominantly Ga (Amanfro), while the sixth is Adangbe (Tubaman). The Ga and Adangbe are usually classified together as Ga-Adangbe due to their very close ethnolinguistic affinity. Ethnolinguistic group essentially determines the dominant lineage rules in each community, which in turn has repercussions for gender relations and other factors bearing on reproductive behavior (Lesthaeghe

1989). Hence the ethnic composition of the communities is a critical element in the argument developed in this chapter.

Table 2.1
Basic Features of the Six Communities

Feature	Abuesi	Amanfro	Brenu-Akyinim	Frami	Kom-foeku	Tubaman
Region	Western	Greater Accra	Central	Central	Western	Greater Accra
Ecology	Coastal	Inland	Coastal	Inland	Inland	Inland
Primary Economic Activity	Fishing	Trading	Farming Fishing	Farming	Farming	Farming
Mean number of household possessions[a]	3.5	4.6	3.4	2.7	3.2	5.0
Percent of households electrified[a]	88	85	71	79	74	82
Percent JSS+ schooling[b]						
Women	27	45	58	49	30	32
Men	32	79	60	77	62	41
Religious Affiliation[c]	OC = 29% PC = 37% M = 24%	OC = 17% PC = 68% M = 7%	OC = 71% PC = 19% M = 2%	OC = 50% PC = 41% M = 0%	OC = 38% PC = 46% M = 0%	OC = 4% PC = 6% M = 90%
Primary Ethno-linguistic Group	Akan	Ga-Adangbe	Akan	Akan	Akan	Ga-Adangbe

Source: Community Portraits; Panel Survey

[a]Calculated for reproductive-age women interviewed in Round 3 of Panel Survey. Adjusted for community differences in age and marital status (through poisson and logit regressions).
[b]JSS+ = junior secondary schooling completed. Calculated for reproductive-age women and their male partners interviewed in Round 1 of Panel Survey. Adjusted for community differences in age and, for women, marital status (through logit regression).
[c]Percentage distribution of reproductive-age women interviewed in Round 1 of Panel Survey. OC = Orthodox Christian; PC = Pentecostal Christian; M = Muslim.

SOCIAL ORGANIZATION

Kinship and Gender Relations

In all these communities, the family, the clan, and the lineage are central to the identity and well-being of the individual. Generally, the Akan communities of Abuesi, Brenu-Akyinim, Frami, and Komfoeku follow the matrilineal inheritance system, while the Ga-Adangbe communities of Amanfro and Tubaman follow the patrilineal system. Yet among the former, certain positions such as *Asafohene*[1] and the chief priests of the gods are inherited patrilineally. Between the two Ga-Adangbe communities, the people of Tubaman stress the principles of patrikin and male dominance more than the people of Amanfro.

In the eyes of the people of Tubaman, a child is first of all a lineage member, and one of the chief purposes of socialization is to produce a loyal and worthy addition to the lineage. The residents of Tubaman, therefore, practice a system of patriarchy and patrilocality (coresidence of husband and wife after marriage) that ensures male dominance over females. Islam reinforces, and supplements, the patrilineal strains in the Ga-Adangbe culture (see Lesthaeghe 1989: 34). In the Community Portrait of Tubaman, it is reported that decision-making about most matters is strictly male-dominated, with the exception of those areas of exclusive concern to women. (For instance, when the women meet alone, as in the 31st December Women's Movement, they are allowed to assume leadership roles.) During worship, only males are allowed to play leadership roles; women are not allowed to stand before men and preach. A ten-year-old boy among a group of elderly women will be the only qualified person to preach, a policy derived directly from Islamic law. In every home the man is supposed to be the head, with the adult women supporting him as deputies, his sons following in authority, and his daughters having the least power.

This male dominance in the family and community in Tubaman contrasts very much with the position of men in the nearby market town of Amanfro and in the four farming and fishing Akan-speaking communities. It is often the practice in Amanfro, as in other Ga-Adangbe communities, that after marriage the husband continues to live in the men's compound of his father and the wife in the women's compound of her mother. Men take their meals together in the men's compound, although the food may have come from wives in several different women's compounds. Under this arrangement, neither partner is under the strict control of the other for most of the day. Not only do these kinship practices of the people of Amanfro have implications for power and authority in marriages (for example, the degree to which the spouses share interests and resources), they also have implications for social interaction patterns: there is less opportunity for exchange of information between spouses and more opportunity for spouses to interact with other persons. In general, Ghanaians interact most frequently with other residents of the same compound (this is documented by the Panel Survey data on social network partners), and hence the traditional Ga-Adangbe residence pattern provides more opportunity for nonspousal social interaction than would be the case were the spouses coresiding. We return to this point below when considering social networks.

However, there is evidence of change in the customary coresidence patterns in Amanfro, suggesting that the pattern of separate residence for spouses may have begun to break down. Today one observes many nuclear-family households composed of a husband, his wife, and their unmarried children. A related feature of the Amanfro traditional family system that seems to be breaking down is the merging of households into a more inclusive segment. Fortes (1949) terms this the "effective minimal lineage." In traditional Ga-Adangbe society, a man had little jural, ritual, and economic authority while his father was alive, because the household of the man and his children was submerged in a more inclusive segment with the man's father as the head. In recent decades, this full merging of households is rare, although most compounds are still headed by the fathers and male elders of the patrilineage. Today the authority of the senior man is more limited in reach, because an increasing fraction of households are organized around the conjugal pair. In Amanfro as compared to Tubaman, women are more able to exert authority in their families by virtue of being the main breadwinners of the household. Unlike Tubaman, in Amanfro decision making is not monopolized by men, despite the fact that the people of Amanfro, like those of Tubaman, are patriarchal in their kinship system and in many practices concerning family matters.

The Akan communities are influenced by an entirely different set of traditional kinship rules. In Akan society descent is primarily matrilineal, although patrilineal descent is the norm for certain positions, for example the *Asafo* executioners (members of the *Asafohene)* and priests. For this reason, some scholars prefer to classify Akan society as based on bilateral descent (e.g., Lesthaeghe 1989: 39). The interplay of these two systems makes for distinctive spousal roles and decision making authority in Akan communities. Wives are expected to reside with their husbands after marriage. This may be neolocal residence, but is often virilocal or patrilocal. The residential arrangement and the matrilineal descent combine to balance spousal relations within marriage. The household organization is centered on the conjugal pair, with the husband normally regarded as the head. Although in this position the husband has some control over the decision making process, he is expected to consult his wife on most family issues, with her views exercising an important influence on the eventual decisions and actions. Hence, while the man is regarded as the ultimate authority, the norms and rules of this system do not nurture overbearing male dominance, instead encourage intensive negotiation and bargaining between spouses.

The links between kinship system and postpartum practices should be noted. In the strict patriarchal system characterizing Tubaman, the new mother does not reside in her kin's home during the postpartum period, rather remains with her husband. In contrast, in the matrilineal system of the Akans, a woman can return to her parental kin during the postpartum period, and indeed births may be delivered away from the husband's compound. The loose patrilineal system of the Ga-Adangbe in Amanfro does not appear to include any hard and fast rules about the location of the woman during pregnancy and the postpartum period, although by the logic of the residential arrangement the new mother would, more often than not, be found in her kin's compound.

Other aspects of kinship that bear directly on reproduction do not vary in their essential features among the six communities. Polygamous marriage is allowed and practiced in all the study communities. In the Panel Survey data, the percentage of women in polygynous unions is as follows, ordered from high to low: Tubaman, 41 percent; Amanfro, 31 percent; Abuesi, 30 percent; Komfoeku, 26 percent; Brenu-Akyinim, 21 percent; Frami, 13 percent. Note that the prevalence of polygamous marriage is somewhat higher in the two Ga-Adangbe communities, which also happen to be somewhat more prosperous, judging by the indicators in Table 2.1. (An additional factor in the case of Tubaman is that Islamic law permits polygyny.) In general in these communities the choice of a mate is not a matter for the individual alone: parents and other senior agnates still exercise some control over matchmaking, for marriage not only unites the couple, it also establishes a new and important relationship between their respective lineages.[2] The primary rationale for marriage is the production of children, and it is the wish of every member of the family and the descent group to carry on the line and to maintain the strength of the lineage and the clan. Thus infertility in particular is frowned upon and puts women at increased risk of divorce or the man taking on another wife. This puts much pressure on women to reproduce, and the Community Portraits describe how women consult herbalists, spiritualists, and priests (traditional) to assist them in conceiving and bearing children.

From the discussion so far, three distinct types of male-female relationships can be discerned in the six communities under study. There is the Tubaman (or islamized) type of male-female relationship, which is characterized by male dominance over the female. This is a relatively extreme case of patriarchal community in the West African setting, and it is tightened by Islamic law. Decision making, both public and private, lies in the hands of men. Farthest from this among the study communities is the type of male-female relationship found in Amanfro. Although descent is reckoned patrilineally, this is not accompanied by a forceful patriarchy. Women are not under the strict control of their husbands, and therefore may take decisions independent of their husbands. It is the relative weakness of the conjugal bond that is the most salient characteristic of this system. The third type of male-female relationship is represented by the Akan bilateral system that is the traditional system in the other four communities. Compared with the male-female relationship among the peoples of Tubaman and Amanfro, the Akan male-female relationship may therefore be described as one of partnership rather than male dominance (Tubaman) or loose relationship (Amanfro).

The classification of the six communities in terms of the gender relations that can be expected to result from the traditional kinship system is as follows:

Community	**Gender Relations**
Abuesi	Complementary
Amanfro	Independence
Brenu-Akyinim	Complementary
Frami	Complementary
Komfoeku	Complementary
Tubaman	Male control

Voluntary Organizations

We now turn to an investigation of the presence of voluntary organizations in the six communities, as measured in the Organization Inventory. It is important to be clear about the purposes of this investigation. Undoubtedly some of the voluntary organizations listed in the Inventory are actively pro- or antinatalist, and this in itself may influence members' reproductive attitudes and behaviors, thereby contributing to differences among the communities in reproductive behavior. For this reason, we take note of what the Organization Inventory indicates about the fertility-related activities of the organizations. However, we regard this evidence as merely suggestive. For one thing, the descriptions in the Organization Inventory of fertility-related activities are brief and selective. Moreover, a thorough investigation of this hypothesized effect of voluntary organizations on reproductive behavior should take account of the intensity of individuals' participation in these organizations. But the Panel Survey does not contain a comprehensive measurement of the respondents' organizational activities. (We hope to rectify this in a future round.) Instead, the main purpose here is to assess how the communities vary in the number of voluntary organizations and their distribution by type (e.g., religious versus political). Of particular concern is how the voluntary organizations might bear on gender systems, as described in the previous section of this chapter, and on patterns of social interaction, to be considered in the next section. In this respect this investigation of voluntary organizations is a bridge between those two discussions, which themselves are central to the argument of this chapter.

We would be remiss not to acknowledge our awareness that local-level organizations have, of late, captured the fancy of many in the field of international development. Taking off from the concept of "social capital" developed by Bourdieu and Coleman in the 1980s (Coleman 1988; Coleman 1990; Bourdieu and Wacquant 1992), the notion that development initiatives are more likely to succeed in those communities that are rich in voluntary organizations has become quite popular. The argument is not that voluntary organizations engage in deliberate activities in support of the development initiatives, although indeed this certainly may occur and contribute to an observed association between community development and organizational density. Rather, the hypothesis is that the social bonds nurtured by voluntary organizations constitute a resource ("social capital") that make communities more receptive to development initiatives and better positioned to maximize their benefit from such initiatives. This is so for multiple reasons, according to social capital theorists, including the social cohesion and trust that voluntary organizations tend to nurture, their capacity to motivate individuals to pursue collective goals rather than private self-interest (which can readily undermine the dividends for all concerned), and, finally, the channels for social diffusion that voluntary organizations provide. It is the latter mechanism that is of particular relevance to this study. In an effort to test the social capital argument, a growing set of empirical studies has related the density of local voluntary organizations to the success of development initiatives (e.g., Narayan and Pritchett 1999). The present study adopts the main hypothesis from social capital theory, i.e., that a larger number of voluntary organizations in a community should be associated, *ceteris paribus*, with more rapid change in health and reproductive behaviors. However, we are mindful of the opposite argument, namely that a higher density of organizations can present an obstacle to change (as pointed out, for example, by Portes and Landolt 1996). Vital and respected organizations and their leaders can promote, but they may also obstruct, the acceptance of innovative ideas, technologies, and behaviors. By constraining the channels for communication, they may accelerate or retard the pace of innovation. Because the social capital effect is not unambiguously unidirectional, it is all the more important to carry out empirical studies of the association between social capital indicators (such as the density of voluntary organizations) and community change (in this instance, adoption of innovative reproductive behaviors).

The Organization Inventory yielded an extensive listing of organizations in each community. For purposes of this chapter, these organizations have been classified under seven categories (Table 2.2): cultural, religious, occupational, political, educational (school-related), philanthropic/welfare, and health/family life education. Several of these major categories have been further divided. Within the religious category, Christian and Moslem organizations are distinguished. (Incidentally, no traditional religious organization was identified in any of the communities, though traditional religious practices are reported in all communities except Tubaman.) The occupational category has been further subclassified into farming, fishing, trading, and others (hairdressers, drivers, etc.). In addition, modern and traditional political organizations are distinguished, to take cognizance of the fact that whereas modern political organizations have nationwide links and functions, traditional political organizations are local institutions. Finally, a distinction between traditional and modern health organizations is drawn, on the assumption that their reproductive health values and practices will often differ, with traditional organizations more likely to be pronatalist and modern health organizations antinatalist.

Counts of the number of each type of organization, by community, are presented in Table 2.2. The number of organizations ranges from a high of twenty-six in Amanfro to a low of eleven in Tubaman.[3] Examination of the distributions by type of organization reveals that the relative shortfall in Tubaman is accounted for mainly by the small number of religious organizations. Religious organizations constitute only about one-quarter of the organizations reported in Tubaman but in the other five communities is by far the most common type. This should not be interpreted as evidence that religion holds less sway over individuals' lives in Tubaman than in the other five communities. On the contrary, as noted earlier Tubaman is a Muslim community, with Islam exerting a dominating influence on their values and practices in all realms of life. Indeed, the Community Portrait states that the people of Tubaman do not admit of values and practices that are contrary to Islamic law. In short, there is less rationale for religious organizations per se in Tubaman, because even without such organizations religion is a pervasive presence in community life. No other community is as religiously homogeneous as Tubaman, as documented in Table 2.1. In the other five communities, therefore, a plethora of religious organizations (as many as sixteen in Komfoeku!) offer community members a means to observe and celebrate with cobelievers their own particular faith.

Table 2.2
Number of Organizations, by Community and Type of Organization

Type of Organization	Abuesi	Amanfro	Brenu-Akyinim	Frami	Kom-foeku	Tuba-man
Cultural	—	1	—	—	—	—
Religious:						
(i) Christian	10	11	8	8	16	—
(ii) Moslem	—	—	—	—	—	3
Occupational:						
(i) Farming	—	—	3	1	1	1
(ii) Fishing	1	—	1	—	—	—
(iii) Trading	—	1	—	—	—	—
(iv) Others	1	3	—	1	1	—
Political:						
(i) Modern	4	3	1	2	2	3
(ii) Traditional	1	1	1	1	2	0
Educational (school-related)	3	4	2	2	1	2
Philanthropic/ Welfare	2	2	—	1	—	2
Health (FLE):						
(i) Traditional	—	—	—	1	—	—
(ii) Modern	1	—	—	—	—	—
Total	23	26	16	17	23	11

Source: Organization Inventory

It is also evident in Table 2.2 that all the communities except Tubaman have a traditional political organization as a complement to the chieftancy system and the modern political organizations (the latter including the unit committee or town development committee, both common in local communities throughout Ghana). One traditional political organization is the *Asafo Company*, found in all sites except Tubaman, which acts as both secular and sacred organization. Members of the *Asafo* are the traditional soldiers of the village, guarding and protecting the people both physically and spiritually. This organization is not present in Tubaman, again reflecting the pervasive influence of Islam in that community.

All six of the communities have educational organizations. The most common are the parent-teacher association (PTA) and the school management committee (SMC). Given the eventual aim of explaining variations in reproductive behavior, gender relations are a major concern of this chapter. The information contained in the Organization Inventory permits classification of the organizations in terms of the gender composition of their membership. Often this is clear from the organization's name: for example, the Jihad Women's Movement, the Assemblies of God Women's Ministry, and the Methodist Women's Fellowship are exclusively for women, whereas both men and women participate in the African Faith Tabernacle, the Methodist Youth Fellowship, and the Catholic Choir. From the membership lists in the Organization Inventory—sometimes complete, but often incomplete—it is also possible to determine whether the membership is of mixed or single gender. On the basis of this information, Table 2.3 has been constructed, which shows the distribution of voluntary organizations according to their gender composition.

The majority of organizations are mixed-gender in all communities except Tubaman, where roughly one-half (five out of eleven) are mixed-gender. In Abuesi, Amanfro, and Frami, about three-quarters of the organizations have both men and women as members. Among the single-gender organizations, female organizations tend to be more common, although once again Tubaman is the exception. In sum, Tubaman is somewhat eccentric, but otherwise the communities resemble each other in the gender composition of their voluntary organizations.

As indicated above, the Organization Inventory contains minimal information on whether or not each organization engages in fertility-related activities. It is plausible that these organizations exercise influence on the views of their members, and hence that organizations whose activities, programs, or objectives include reproductive ideas and behavior would have an impact on the reproductive attitudes and behavior of their members. This effect might be positive or negative, depending on the messages conveyed by the organization. As it happens, organizations reported in the Organization Inventory are primarily antinatalist in their emphasis, which itself may be revealing of a less than comprehensive measurement of the full range of relevant activities.

For now, we simply count the number of organizations that have fertility-related programs or objectives. The counts are as follows: Komfoeku, 5 (out of 23); Abuesi, 4 (out of 23); Amanfro, 1 (out of 26); Frami, 1 (out of 17); Brenu-Akyinim, 0 (out of 16); Tubaman, 0 (out of 11). It is, then, a small minority of organizations for which such activities are reported. Of the four organizations in Abuesi, two are women's Christian groups, one is a mixed-gender Christian

Table 2.3
Number of Organizations, by Community, Gender Composition, and Type of Organization

Type of Organization	Abuesi			Amanfro			Brenu-Akyinim			Frami			Komfoeku			Tubaman		
	Gender of Membership of Organization[a]																	
	M	F	X	M	F	X	M	F	X	M	F	X	M	F	X	M	F	X
Cultural	—	—	—	—	—	1	—	—	—	—	—	—	—	—	—	—	—	—
Religious:																		
(i) Christian	—	3	7	—	2	9	—	3	5	—	2	6	1	6	9	—	—	—
(ii) Moslem	—	—	—	—	—	—	—	—	—	—	—	—	—	—	—	—	1	2
Occupational:																		
(i) Farming	—	—	—	—	—	—	1	—	2	—	—	1	1	—	—	1	—	—
(ii) Fishing	1	—	—	—	—	—	—	—	1	—	—	—	—	—	—	—	—	—
(iii) Trading	—	—	—	—	1	—	—	—	—	—	—	—	—	—	—	—	—	—
(iv) Others	1	—	—	—	—	3	—	—	—	—	—	1	1	—	—	—	—	—
Political:																		
(i) Modern	—	—	4	—	1	2	—	—	1	—	—	1	—	1	1	1	1	1
(ii) Traditional	—	—	1	1	—	—	1	—	—	—	1	1	1	—	1	—	—	—
Educational (school-related)	—	—	3	—	—	4	—	—	2	—	—	2	—	—	1	1	—	1
Philanthropic/ Welfare	1	—	1	—	—	2	—	—	—	—	—	1	—	—	—	1	—	1
Health (FLE[b]*):*																		
(i) Traditional	—	—	—	—	—	—	—	—	—	—	1	—	—	—	—	—	—	—
(ii) Modern	—	—	1	—	—	—	—	—	—	—	—	—	—	—	—	—	—	—
Total	3	3	17	1	4	21	2	3	11	—	4	13	4	7	12	4	2	5
%	13	13	74	4	15	81	12	19	69	—	23	77	18	30	52	36	18	46

Source: Organization Inventory
[a] "M" denotes male, "F" denotes female, "X" denotes mixed gender.
[b] "FLE" refers to "family life education."

group, and the fourth is a mixed-gender modern health/family life education club. The five organizations in Komfoeku are all Christian organizations, with four being women's groups and the fifth a mixed-gender group. Clearly, the common belief that religious organizations are less likely to promote antinatalist than pronatalist attitudes and behaviors is not borne out by the information in the Organization Inventory.

Summing up, the following points have emerged from this investigation of voluntary organizations. First, the organizations are numerous, with only Tubaman lagging in its density of organizations. Second, religious organizations are most common, followed by political organizations. Third, the majority of these organizations have mixed-gender membership. Fourth, only a few of the organizations have activities, programs, or objectives that aim at educating or influencing their members about reproductive behavior.

PATTERNS OF SOCIAL INTERACTION

The second major research tradition informing this chapter is the literature on social diffusion. According to the theory and empirical studies in this tradition, one process through which social change occurs is the diffusion of ideas, technologies, and behaviors from one social group to another (Rogers 1983). There are various channels for social diffusion, including the mass media, agents of organized interventions (school teachers, health workers, Christian missionaries), and, of most concern in this analysis, informal social interaction. The hypothesis is that through informal social interaction—with kin, neighbors, friends, workmates—women and men are exposed to new reproductive attitudes and practices (Montgomery and Casterline 1998, Casterline 2001b). The extent of such exposure, in turn, is a function of individuals' social interaction patterns, and more specifically what are commonly termed "social networks."

In southern Ghana at the present time, it is plausible that the key issue concerning social networks, from the standpoint of their efficacy in facilitating (or hindering) the social diffusion of innovative reproductive attitudes and behaviors, is the extent to which they expose individuals to persons from a diversity of social groups (as defined by ethnicity, religion, educational attainment, social class, age, and so forth). Of particular significance is whether individuals social networks contain persons outside the community, thereby providing a channel for innovative ideas and behaviors to enter the community. Following established theory on social diffusion (with roots in Granovetter's seminal 1973 article), we distinguish "heterogeneous" from "homogeneous" networks, the former being diverse in their membership (in terms of basic social attributes) and the latter less diverse. Homogeneous networks are assumed to be more insulated and more likely to support prevailing social norms and practices than to challenge them. In contrast, heterogeneous networks are more likely to offer their members an opportunity to consider a wider range of options for their personal behavior and a reduced pressure to conform to prevailing community norms. In short, heterogeneous networks are more likely to promote social diffusion (Watkins 1991; Kohler et al. 2001).

To this basic hypothesis, which is appealing in its logic and simplicity, an important qualification must be added (Valente 1995). The hypothesis as stated explains why innovations might enter some communities more easily, and sooner, than other communities. The initial introduction of an innovation can be viewed as the first stage of social diffusion, and perhaps is the primary determinant of the overall pace of social change in a society. However, the rapidity with which an innovation spreads *within* a community is another matter. Within-community diffusion should be more rapid where the patterns of within-community communication are such that a large fraction of members soon learn about the innovation, and where social norms can more quickly adapt to the new ideas, technologies, or behaviors. It is plausible that social interaction patterns in homogeneous communities, rather than heterogeneous communities, are more conducive to within-community social diffusion (Valente 1995; Casterline 2001a). The more constraining social pressure assumed to be characteristic of homogeneous communities can obstruct social change, but ironically it can also facilitate social change. A more elaborate hypothesis, then, is that innovations gain a foothold sooner in heterogeneous communities, but once established accumulate adherents at a more rapid pace in homogeneous communities. If, then, one is examining the prevalence of innovative attitudes and behaviors—modern contraception, for example—it is not entirely clear whether at any particular historical date the prevalence should be higher or lower in heterogeneous as compared to homogeneous communities.

For this analysis, we favor the basic network-type hypothesis, i.e., that heterogeneous social networks are more conducive to social diffusion. The primary justification for retaining this basic hypothesis is that in southern Ghana reproductive decisions appear to be regarded as essentially private matters, almost entirely within the province of reproductive-age couples and their immediate kin. Hence there would appear to be less potential for the positive reinforcement of innovative decisions that homogeneous communities can more effectively offer. However, social norms and pressures are by no means irrelevant in this setting, and we will remain mindful of the qualification articulated in the previous paragraph. As it will turn out, this qualification will assist our interpretation of some cross-community variation in innovative reproductive behavior that is otherwise quite puzzling.

The task now is to characterize the six study communities in terms of patterns of social interaction, that is, the typical structure of social networks, separately for men and for women. To this end, three clusters of variables are considered: (1) gender systems and male-female relationships (described earlier in this chapter); (2) the nature of economic activity in each of the communities (described in the Community Portraits), under the assumption that economic activity is a primary factor structuring patterns of social interaction (especially extra-community interaction); and (3) individuals' geographic mobility and social networks (measured in the Panel Survey).

Beginning with gender systems and their hypothesized effects on network types, these have far more bearing on the social networks of women than of men, because none of the systems constrain men to any meaningful extent.

Everything else being equal, women's social networks should be relatively heterogeneous in communities characterized by gender independence, as in the Ga-Adangbe patrilineal system found in Amanfro. Women in Amanfro need not ask for permission or concurrence of their spouses when making decisions, even if those decisions have implications for the immediate family. Less heterogeneous, but still placing relatively limited constraints on women, is the system of "complementary" gender relations found in the Akan communities (Abuesi, Brenu-Akyinim, Frami, and Komfoeku), with their bilateral reckoning of descent. Finally, in Tubaman, with its strongly patriarchal kinship system and male-controlled gender relations, women are least free to circulate and form social relationships of their own choosing, and hence social networks are expected to be relatively homogeneous. However, because of the hierarchical decision making power wielded by men in Tubaman, the qualification to the network-type hypothesis noted above—that within-community social diffusion can occur more rapidly in tightly knit communities—may well apply to Tubaman. In short, the implications of the gender systems for the women's social networks are clear: the most heterogeneous networks are in Amanfro, the most homogeneous are in Tubaman, and the Akan communities fall somewhere in between.

Turning to economic activity, there is substantial diversity among the six communities in the prevailing types of economic activities and the extent to which these encourage social mixing. We devote some space to a description of the principal economic activities in each community and the implications for social networks. Because of the predominance of trading in Amanfro, the men and women of this community are likely to have more contact with persons outside the community than residents of any of the other five communities. In particular, the women of Amanfro trade at nearby Kasoa and the more distant Mankesim markets, both of which are on the main Accra–Cape Coast trunk road and attract people from several regions of the country. They also trade in Accra. The daily commuting of the residents of Amanfro between Kasoa, Mankesim, and Accra exposes them to diverse groups of people and information. Indeed, the Community Portrait for Amanfro notes that Amanfro traders have received information about modern contraception from market conversations with other traders and conversations with "self-proclaimed doctors" and "nurses" who come to the market to sell drugs, including contraceptives.

The residents of Tubaman, like those of Amanfro, also engage in trade. In contrast to Amanfro, however, agriculture is the main source of livelihood for households in Tubaman. The norm is for a husband and wife to farm together, and for the woman to perform the additional task of selling the produce. Marketing the produce brings the women of Tubaman into contact with other farmers and residents of the nearby market town of Kasoa, and Accra as well. For this reason, the extracommunity social exposure of Tubaman women may approach that of Amanfro women, despite the Islamic norm of social seclusion of women. If economic activity were the only criterion, then one might posit that the social networks of Tubaman residents are nearly as heterogeneous as those of Amanfro residents.

The economic activities of the residents of Frami and Komfoeku force far less extracommunity social interaction. As in Tubaman, the main occupation in these communities is farming, but a larger fraction is subsistence farming, i.e., for household use with no marketing of farm goods. Wives in particular do not travel regularly to markets and receive cash from sales of produce, rather their husbands give them farm produce that they process for domestic use and for limited sales activity in the community. Much of this will be traded using the barter system, with food items like gari, kenkey, and edible oil exchanged for cassava, corn, and coconut. There is very little money in the system and, for that matter, there is very little exchange and contact between the people and the outside world. This system of economic activity on balance nurtures homogeneous social networks.

The story is much the same for Brenu-Akyinim, although the economic activity there is not as self-contained within the community as is the case in Frami and Komfoeku. Brenu-Akyinim is a coastal settlement, with farming and salt winning (salt mining) being the leading economic activities. A minority of Ewe migrants engages in fishing. The farmers engage in subsistence farming, grow food for home consumption, but also grow cash crops for marketing (maize, cassava, plantain, tomatoes, tiger nut, and coconut). The women engage in food preparation and the sale of salt and pineapple. Recently there has been an effort to promote pineapple production for export. In short, economic activities in Brenu-Akyinim provide the community residents with some limited social interaction with persons from outside the community.

While both Brenu Akyinim and Abuesi are coastal settlements, only in Abuesi is fishing the main economic activity. The men catch the fish, and the women are fish smokers and/or fish mongers. This brings the women into contact with persons from other communities, especially women who come to the community to buy fish or whom they meet in the market in nearby communities or occasionally in more distant cities (Sekondi-Takoradi and Cape Coast). In addition to the fish industry, Abuesi has been introduced to new economic activities and extracommunity social interaction as a result of the construction and installation of the thermal plant in the adjacent town of Aboadzi. One can find in Abuesi a wide range of economic activities, including carpentry, blacksmithing, dressmaking, hairdressing, and food preparation. Economic activity in Abuesi, hence, leads to more heterogeneous social networks than in the other three Akan communities (Brenu-Akyinim, Frami, Komfoeku).

We conclude this section by examining Panel Survey data on geographic mobility and social networks (Table 2.4). Two indicators of geographic mobility are presented: the percentage of respondents born in the community, and the percentage who visited a city (Accra, Kumasi, Takoradi, or Cape Coast) at least once per month on average since the previous interview (six to nine months for most respondents). Roughly one-half of the respondents in the four Akan communities (Abuesi, Brenu-Akyinim, Frami, and Komfoeku) were born in that community. The fraction is slightly more than one-third in Tubaman, and only one-eighth in Amanfro. Judging from this indicator, the Akan communities are far more insulated than the two Ga-Adangbe communities, Amanfro in particu-

Table 2.4
Indicators of Geographic Mobility, Mass Media Exposure, and Social Interaction Patterns, by Community[a]

Variables[b]	Abuesi	Amanfro	Brenu-Akyinim	Frami	Komfoeku	Tubaman
Percent born in the community [R1, W]	50	12	52	51	58	38
Percent visit cities[c] once/month or more often since last interview [R2]						
Women	20	80	35	47	40	50
Men	41	89	57	58	77	71
Percent watch television twice/week or more often since last interview [R2]						
Women	35	71	42	41	36	37
Men	50	79	46	44	51	53
Percent informal discussions about AIDS since last interview [R2]						
Women	15	66	19	55	16	16
Men	35	83	32	66	35	30
Mean number of network partners:						
Discuss important matters [R1]						
Women	4.1	3.4	3.5	3.5	2.8	4.1
Men	4.8	4.2	4.2	3.9	3.0	4.5
Discuss modern contraception [R2]						
Women	1.2	2.2	1.4	1.9	0.9	1.7
Men	1.4	2.4	1.7	2.3	1.2	1.5
Discuss HIV/AIDS [R3]						
Women	1.5	1.4	0.9	1.6	0.6	1.2
Men	1.9	2.2	1.1	1.7	0.9	1.6

Source: Panel Survey. Sample is limited to women interviewed in Round 1. Round 3 estimates, for example, are based on respondents also interviewed in Round 1. The men are partners of women interviewed in Round 1.

[a]All differentials across communities are adjusted for community differences in age and, for women, marital status. The adjustments are carried out through fitting logit or poisson regressions. The statistical significance of variation among communities in each measure has been tested; for all measures shown, the variation among communities is significant at the .001 level.

[b]R1, R2, R3 denote Panel Survey Rounds 1, 2, and 3, respectively. W and M denote women and men samples, respectively.

[c]Accra, Kumasi, Takoradi, Cape Coast.

lar. Amanfro also is distinctive in the intensity of recent circulation to cities: 80 percent of Amanfro women visit cities at least once per month, whereas the corresponding figure is 50 percent for Tubaman women and lower yet for women in the four Akan communities (nearly 50 percent in Frami, which has easy access via a main road to Cape Coast, and as low as 20 percent in Abuesi, despite its relative proximity to Takoradi). The pattern for men is essentially the same, with Amanfro men most likely to have visited cities (almost 90 percent) and Abuesi men least likely (about 40 percent).

Frequent television viewing (at least twice per week on average) is substantially more likely in Amanfro, for both women and men (third panel of Table 2.4). There is little variation among the other five communities in this indicator of mass media exposure.

It is possible that the majority of the residents of these communities were unaware of HIV/AIDS when this research project was initiated in the early 1990s. We have no data to confirm or refute this suspicion, but Panel Survey data collected in 1998 show that awareness of this disease was almost universal by that date—hardly surprising, given the proliferation in the mass media (radio, television, billboards) in the late 1990s of advertisements warning of the disease and promoting risk-avoidance behaviors. Informal discussion has also undoubtedly contributed to the spread of awareness of the disease and modes of infection, and one can view the amount of informal discussion about AIDS as an indicator of the extent to which personal networks are a mechanism for the diffusion of new knowledge and attitudes about health behaviors (fourth panel of Table 2.4). Judging from the frequency of discussion about AIDS, once again the conclusion is that Amanfro is most exposed to outside influences. Frami follows next, with discussion distinctly less common than in Amanfro but substantially more common than in the other four communities, where discussion is far less likely (with no perceptible differences among the four). In all six communities, men are far more likely than women to report having had conversations about AIDS.

Finally, the Panel Survey contains detailed measurements of social networks (fifth panel of Table 2.4). These are conversational networks, defined with reference to different topics in each of the first three rounds of the Panel Survey: important matters (Round 1), modern contraception (Round 2), and HIV/AIDS (Round 3). Respondents in Komfoeku report the smallest number of conversational partners for all three topics. The communities that rank high, however, vary according to topic: Abuesi and Tubaman for important matters, Amanfro for modern contraception, and Amanfro and Abuesi (and, for women, Frami) for HIV/AIDS. The picture is cloudy, but one might conclude that on average conversational networks are somewhat larger in Amanfro and Abuesi and smaller in Komfoeku. On the whole these differentials are consistent with other features of the communities, although it is a bit surprising that conversational networks are not relatively larger in Brenu-Akyinim, given the patterns of economic activity and the nearby beach resort, quite popular with Ghanaian and international tourists.

What can be concluded about community differences in typical social networks? It is difficult to settle on simple characterizations, because the various pieces of information examined here imply somewhat different rankings of the communities. Moreover, in some instances these rankings vary by gender. Even allowing for this complexity, however, it is clear that the empirical data in hand suggest that social networks are most heterogeneous in the market town Amanfro—this is the least ambiguous inference—and on balance more homogeneous in the farming communities of Frami and Komfoeku. Abuesi, Brenu-Akyinim, and Tubaman fall somewhere in between, with the networks possibly more heterogeneous in Abuesi than in Brenu and Tubaman. In short, Amanfro stands out as unique, and for women in particular, because of their exposure to a diversity of individuals in the market and the rather limited male constraints on their day-to-day mobility.

From this discussion emerges the following classification of the six communities in terms of the heterogeneity/homogeneity of social networks:

Community	**Type of Social Network**
Abuesi	Heterogeneous
Amanfro	Highly heterogeneous
Brenu-Akyinim	Somewhat homogeneous
Frami	Homogeneous
Komfoeku	Homogeneous
Tubaman	Somewhat heterogeneous

REPRODUCTIVE BEHAVIOR

We now examine differentials among the communities in reproductive behavior, as calculated from the Panel Survey (Table 2.5). Three different aspects of reproduction are considered: actual fertility, as indicated by the cumulative number of live births; the main proximate determinants of fertility, specifically nuptiality, postpartum practices (breast feeding, abstinence), and contraception; and, fertility desires. As argued in the first section of this chapter, fertility is in the process of decline in Ghana, probably indicative of a decrease in the number of children desired. The primary direct cause of the fertility decline to date, in particular the decline during the 1990s, is increased practice of contraception (Ghana Statistical Service and Macro International 1999; Blanc and Grey 2000).

In thinking about differences in reproductive behavior among the six communities, it is certainly possible that there have been differences in marriage and postpartum practices in the past that have persisted to the present and that might lead to intercommunity differences in fertility rates. Of more interest at this historical juncture, however, are differences in *fertility desires* and in the *practice of contraception* (modern methods in particular), because these are indicative of communities' participation in the ongoing fertility transition in Ghana. It is, of course, with this priority in mind that previous sections of this chapter

Table 2.5
Indicators of Reproductive Behavior, by Community

Variables	Abuesi	Amanfro	Brenu-Akyinim	Frami	Komfoeku	Tubaman	Significance[a]
Children ever born[b]							
Women	4.1	3.5	3.9	3.9	4.1	4.2	*
Men[c]	6.5	4.4	5.2	4.6	5.2	6.5	**
Median age at first marriage							
Women	19.8	20.2	20.1	20.3	20.4	20.2	-
Men	22.0	24.8	25.9	25.6	25.6	25.7	-
Breast feeding: percent still breast feeding at 24 months postpartum							
Women	26	20	32	34	31	40	n.s.
Postpartum abstinence: percent abstaining at 6 months postpartum							
Women	67	55	58	36	48	32	**
Percent want no more births[d]							
Women (at 4 living children)	66	55	68	57	55	41	**
Men (at 5 living children)	62	44	52	51	56	36	*
Percent currently using modern method[e] *of contraception*[f]							
Women	12	20	16	28	9	22	**
Men	18	28	23	38	19	31	**
Number of cases[g]							
Women	232	142	171	190	198	175	
Men	153	79	93	109	140	103	

Source: Panel Survey (Round 1, except where otherwise noted).
[a] * denotes significant at .05 level, ** denotes significant at .001 level, n.s. denotes not significant.
[b] Adjusted for community differences in age. The adjustments are carried out through fitting a poisson regression.
[c] Total births fathered, all partners.
[d] Fitted percentages, from logit regressions with living children and living children squared. Average of percentages for Rounds 1–3.
[e] Pill, injection, diaphragm/foam, condom, IUD, ligation, Norplant.
[f] Adjusted for community differences in age. The adjustments are carried out through fitting logit regressions. Average of percentages for Rounds 1–3.
[g] Round 1 respondents. Ever-married women. Men are current partners of women in sample.

concentrated on social organizational features that might hinder or facilitate the social diffusion of innovative ideas, technologies, and behaviors.

Before examining community differences in fertility desires and contraceptive practice, we briefly review differentials in actual fertility, marriage, and postpartum practices (first four panels of Table 2.5). The number of children ever born is calculated for both women and their male partners. Through multiple wives (serially or simultaneously), men on average have one or two more children than do women. As expected, this gender difference tends to be larger where polygyny is more common (Tubaman, and also Abuesi) and smaller where polygyny is less common (Frami); Amanfro, where polygyny is relatively common, runs counter to this expectation. Nevertheless, the pattern of community differentials is essentially the same for women and men: fertility is lowest in Amanfro, and highest in Abuesi and Tubaman.

Because the practice of contraception has not been widespread in these communities in the past, the observed differences in fertility can be attributed to differences in nuptiality and postpartum practices. Interestingly, the timing of entrance to first marriage hardly differs among the six communities (second panel of Table 2.5): women, and especially men, marry earlier in the fishing community of Abuesi, but in the other five communities marry at about the same average age—slightly over age twenty for women, and around age twenty-five for men. Hence nuptiality patterns in the past do not appear to have contributed to community differences in actual fertility. More intercommunity variation is evident for postpartum practices: breast feeding (third panel) and abstinence (fourth panel). The average breast feeding duration is longest in Tubaman, followed by the three Akan farming communities of Frami, Brenu-Akyinim, and Komfoeku, and shortest in Amanfro and Abuesi. Community differentials in postpartum abstinence, which in these communities probably has more impact than breast feeding on fertility levels, follow a different pattern. At six months postpartum, roughly two-thirds of the women are still abstaining in Abuesi, nearly 60 percent in Brenu-Akyinim and Amanfro, roughly one-half in Komfoeku, and only one-third in Frami and Tubaman. The variation across communities in this indicator is surprisingly large. It is difficult, on the basis of this quick overview of selected indicators, to determine how the various proximate determinants, measured and unmeasured (induced abortion), jointly account for observed differences among the communities in the average number of births.

Of more central concern in this research are community differences in childbearing desires and contraceptive practice. We have hypothesized that these facets of reproductive behavior, which are likely to be especially sensitive to the spread of new ideas and behaviors, should be associated with the social organizational features of the communities. The indicator of fertility desires chosen for this analysis is the percentage of respondents who wish to terminate childbearing, shown separately for men and women (fifth panel of Table 2.5). This desire is evaluated at four living children for women and at five living children for men. For contraception, the indicator is the percentage using modern methods, shown separately for men and women (sixth panel of Table 2.5). Because use of modern contraception is the clearly innovative behavior in this setting, as well as being the principal mechanism of the ongoing fertility transition in Ghana, community differentials in this facet of reproductive behavior are of particular interest.

The pattern of community differentials in the fifth and six panels of Table 2.5 varies a bit by gender. Giving more weight to women, we propose the following ranking of the six communities according to fertility desires and use of modern contraception:

Community	Desire to Limit Births	Use of Modern Contraception
Abuesi	High	Low
Amanfro	Moderate	Moderate
Brenu-Akyinim	High	Moderate
Frami	Moderate	High
Komfoeku	Moderate	Low
Tubaman	Low	Moderate

It is surprising that the rankings are so different for fertility desires and contraceptive use. Among other things, this may reflect the fact that much of the contraceptive use is for birth spacing, rather than to terminate childbearing. Even so, it is curious that the relatively high desire to limit births in Abuesi is accompanied by relatively low prevalence of modern contraception (suggestive of relatively high unmet need for family planning in that community), and that contraceptive prevalence is moderately high in Tubaman despite the relatively weak desire to restrict fertility. Contraceptive prevalence is highest in Frami—over one-quarter of women report that they are currently using a modern method—followed by Tubaman and then Amanfro. At the other end, the lowest contraceptive prevalence is found in Komfoeku, followed closely by Abuesi.

PUTTING THE PIECES TOGETHER

The overarching objective of this research is to examine the association between social organization and fertility, through analysis of covariation at the community level in six communities in southern Ghana. We have considered multiple aspects of the social organization (kinship systems, gender relations, social interaction patterns) and juxtaposed them with survey estimates of various reproductive behaviors, focusing on those behaviors thought to be driving the ongoing decline in fertility in Ghana (fertility desires and contraceptive use). As it happens, different aspects of the social organization lead to different expectations about how reproductive behavior should vary among the communities. And, adding further to the challenge of drawing clear conclusions from this analysis, the patterns of reproductive differentials vary depending on the reproductive indicator chosen.

Mindful of these complexities, we arrive at the following summary of our separate analyses of social organization and reproductive behavior. We show community differentials in patterns of both desired fertility and use of modern contraception, since the two patterns are markedly different. The fertility indicators are expressed in terms of their association with the level of fertility; i.e., a high prevalence of desires to stop childbearing and a high prevalence of contraception are both labeled "low" because they should translate into relatively low levels of fertility.

Community	**Expected Fertility Levels Based on Social Organization**	**Observed Fertility Patterns**[a] **(Fertility desires/ Contraceptive use)**
Abuesi	Moderate	Low/High
Amanfro	Low	Moderate/Moderate
Brenu-Akyinim	Moderate	Low/Moderate
Frami	High	Moderate/Low
Komfoeku	High	Moderate/High
Tubaman	Moderate	High/Moderate

[a]The levels refer to fertility desires and use of modern contraception, respectively. They are formulated in terms of effects on fertility levels: "high" refers to low percentages wanting to stop childbearing or using contraception, whereas "low" refers to high percentages wanting to stop childbearing or using contraception.

The fit between expected and observed fertility is disappointing. We expected Amanfro to be most advanced in the fertility transition, as reflected in fertility desires and contraceptive practice, but instead it falls somewhere in the middle among the six communities. (Interestingly, in Table 2.5 Amanfro does show the lowest level of actual fertility, a ranking more consistent with our expectations.) Similarly, Frami and Komfoeku were expected to be less advanced in the fertility transition, and although Komfoeku essentially fulfills this expectation, Frami has a high prevalence of use of modern contraception. Abuesi and Tubaman further confuse the picture: both were expected to show relatively moderate levels of fertility, but this expectation is fulfilled only with respect to modern contraceptive use in Tubaman.

We believe that this unexpected pattern of intercommunity differences in reproductive behavior can be explained, but doing so requires introducing two additional types of information, namely the actions of community leaders and the provision of health and family planning services. Neither of these has figured prominently in our discussion thus far, but they can do much to unravel the mystery of the community differentials in fertility. The major anomalies in the differentials are that contraceptive use is relatively high in relation to expectations in Frami and Tubaman, and relatively low in Amanfro. A reading of the Community Portraits suggest that, in the case of Frami, the explanation may lie in the relatively greater availability of family planning and health services. Frami has a well-functioning health clinic and a drugstore that sells medicines, including contraceptives. In addition, Frami is visited frequently by staff of the Planned Parenthood Association of Ghana (PPAG), as well as government and health personnel from Cape Coast, only thirty-five kilometres away on a major road. Finally, community residents tell of the Frami resident who was sponsored by the village in the early 1990s to undertake formal training in family planning offered by PPAG. The man in question was a member of the town development committee. Since then, he has been organizing family planning discussions with households in the community. These discussions were referred to during focus group discussions conducted in the pilot stage of our project. In short, among the six communities, Frami is perhaps most richly endowed with health and family planning services, and this might well account for its relatively high prevalence of contraceptive use.

The case of Tubaman is even more interesting. The notion of practicing family planning through use of modern contraceptives is relatively new in the community, and is traced by community residents to a specific historical development. Contraception had been regarded as contrary to Islamic teachings. But the present chief's sister's son traveled to Saudi Arabia for his university education, and then returned to Ghana with the news that family planning is compatible with Islam. This was a watershed event. Henceforth family planning could be discussed openly in Tubaman, and contraceptive practice need not be covert. Given the strongly hierarchical structure of social life in Tubaman, this sanctioning of family planning by senior leaders of the community had a larger impact than in most Ghanaian communities. This fits with the argument made earlier in this chapter that homogeneous communities can be conducive to rapid diffusion of innovative behaviors, because social pressure can be exerted more effectively in such communities (with the pressure in this instance coming from community leaders via the strongly hierarchical power structure of the community). Complementing this factor has been the fairly effective provision of health and family-planning services in Tubaman by the health nurse, who holds a weekly Friday clinic in the community. In qualitative interviews, residents tell of women taking their children with them to the Friday clinic, ostensibly to receive medical care for the children but in fact for the purpose of receiving a contraceptive injection.

Finally we consider the case of Amanfro. The relatively low level of contraceptive practice in Amanfro, as compared to our expectations, remains something of a puzzle. We note in Table 2.5 the relative absence of desires to terminate childbearing, suggesting that children are valued somewhat more highly in Amanfro than in some of the other communities. One can argue that, among the various ethnic groups in Ghana, the Ga are relatively more pronatalist, with customary practices that encourage Ga women to bear many children being more strongly maintained than is the case in other ethnic groups. Various initiation rites promote early age at first birth and adolescent pregnancy. While the people of Amanfro regard this as a period of economic hardship and certainly admit the potential economic costs of having a large number of children, the view persists that large numbers of children are an economic asset in old age. This attachment to childbearing, despite its recognized economic costs (and despite the relatively easy and inexpensive availability of contraceptive methods in the community), perhaps explains why contraceptive prevalence is lower in

Amanfro than we predicted. This is largely speculation, and clearly further empirical investigation would be required to verify this explanation.

CONCLUDING REMARKS

The overarching objective of this research has been to examine the association between social organization and reproductive behavior. In contrast to most prior research on sub-Saharan African societies with the same objective (e.g., Lesthaeghe 1989), we have not focused on those aspects of social organization thought to account for societal variation in pretransition reproductive regimes. Pretransition variation in fertility was probably due primarily to nuptiality and postpartum practices. Rather, our concern is how social organization affects the diffusion of innovative reproductive ideas and behaviors. Social diffusion is assumed to be strongly affected by the nature of social interaction patterns, and these in turn are assumed to be determined in part by the social organization of local communities: gender relations, employment activity, and the prominence of voluntary organizations. With this theoretical orientation, we are able to develop explicit hypotheses about how the adoption of fertility control desires and behaviors (e.g., modern contraception) should vary among six communities in southern Ghana.

In the event, the empirical data on fertility obtained in the panel survey does not clearly confirm the hypotheses. This outcome is a disappointment, but we do not regard it as a decisive rejection of the social organization and social diffusion argument. Rather, our conclusion is that research such as this that examines a small number of communities must be sensitive to the particularities and idiosyncrasities of the communities. Two of the study communities—Frami and Tubaman—show relatively high prevalence of contraceptive use, contrary to expectations, and this can be explained by circumstances specific to the recent history of each community (the actions of health workers in both communities, the formal discussions organized by the PPAG-trained man in Frami, and the endorsement of family planning by the religious leadership in Tubaman). Another community—Amanfro—shows lower-than-expected prevalence of contraceptive use, and this may be explained by the continued attachment to pronatalist customary beliefs and practices. A statistical demographer might view this as a "small sample" problem: when the sample consists of merely six communities, historical circumstances specific to one or two communities can leave a strong impression on the results.

A general conclusion is that an explanatory framework that places social organization on center stage must be enlarged to incorporate the potentially powerful influence of community history. In the case of reproductive behavior at times of transition, the history of health and family planning provision can be especially influential in determining whether change starts relatively early or relatively late and whether change proceeds rapidly or slowly. The placement of health and family planning services is the outcome of an altogether different set of forces, following a logic that is primarily political and bureaucratic and that may have little to do with community social organization. Hence when considering the intercommunity pattern of diffusion of new fertility regulation practices, account must be taken of both local social organization and the history of service provision. This general conclusion—that explanatory theory must balance social organization with historical circumstances—emerges from our analysis of variation among small localities. We suspect, however, that the same conclusion applies to comparative historical research on fertility transition at the level of the nation-state. Undoubtedly variables such as mortality decline, schooling, and income are determinants of the timing and pace of fertility transition; these occupy the place of social organization in this analysis. But the stance of political leaders and the effectiveness of health and family planning programs may have substantial bearing on whether transition starts early or late, and whether it proceeds slowly or rapidly.

NOTES

This chapter draws on materials collected under the project "Diffusion of Fertility Behavior," which is a collaboration between the University of Cape Coast (Ghana) and the Population Council (U.S.). The project is supported by awards from the Rockefeller Foundation and the National Institutes of Health (R01 HD34524).

1. The *Asafohene* are the heads of the traditional army, organized to defend the chiefs and community members against external aggression.

2. Discussion of the age at entry to marriage is deferred until the section on community variation in reproductive behavior, because the timing of marriage is an important direct determinant of fertility levels.

3. To give some rough notion of the density of organizations, the population sizes of the six communities according to the census that we carried out in 1998 were as follows: Abuesi = 2494; Amanfro = 858; Brenu = 1211; Frami = 1226; Komfoeku = 2106; Tubaman = 1159. The relatively larger number of organizations in Abuesi and Komfoeku (Table 2.2) is to be expected, given their far larger population sizes. Perhaps most striking is the large number of organizations in Amanfro in relation to its population size.

REFERENCES

Blanc, Ann K., and Steve Grey. (2000). *Greater than Expected Fertility Decline in Ghana: An Examination of the Evidence*. Calverton, MD: Macro International Inc. and National Population Council Secretariat (Ghana).

Bourdieu, Pierre, and Loic Wacquant. (1992). *An Invitation to Reflexive Sociology*. Chicago: University of Chicago Press.

Caldwell, John C. (1982). *Theory of Fertility Decline*. New York: Academic Press.

Casterline, John B. (2001a). The pace of fertility transition: national patterns in the second half of the twentieth century. In R. Bulatao and J. Casterline (eds.). *Global Fertility Transition*. Supplement to *Population and Development Review* 27.

———. (2001b). Introduction. In J. Casterline and B. Cohen (eds.). *Diffusion Processes and Fertility Transition*. Washington, D.C.: National Academy Press.

Coleman, James S. (1988). Social capital in the creation of human capital. *American Journal of Sociology* 94: S95–S120.

———. (1990). *Foundations of Social Theory*. Cambridge, MA: Harvard University Press.

Fortes, Meyer. (1949). *The Web of Kinship among the Tallensi*. London: Oxford University Press.

Ghana Statistical Service (GSS) and Macro International (MI). (1999). *1998 Ghana Demographic and Health Survey*. Calverton, MD: GSS and MI.

Granovetter. (1973). The strength of weak ties. *American Journal of Sociology* 78(6): 1360–1380.

Kohler, Hans Peter, Jere R. Behrman, and Susan C. Watkins. (2001). The density of social networks and fertility decisions: evidence from South Nyanza District, Kenya. *Demography* 38(1): 43–58.

Lesthaeghe, Ron J. (ed.). (1989). *Reproduction and Social Organization in sub-Saharan Africa*. Berkeley: University of California Press.

Lorimer, Frank. (1954). *Culture and Human Fertility—A Study of the Relation of Cultural Conditions to Fertility in Non-industrial and Transitional Societies*. Paris: UNESCO.

Montgomery, Mark R., and John B. Casterline. (1998). Social networks and the diffusion of fertility control. *Policy Research Division Working Paper* no. 119. New York: Population Council.

Narayan, Deepa, and Lant Pritchett. (1999). Cents and sociability: household income and social capital in rural Tanzania. *Economic Development and Cultural Change* 47(4): 871–898.

National Research Council. (1993). *Factors Affecting Contraceptive Use in Sub-Saharan Africa*. Washington, D.C.: National Academy Press.

Portes, Alejandro, and Patricia Landolt. (1996). The downside of social capital. *American Prospect* (May–June): 18–21, 94.

Rogers, Everett M. (1983). *Diffusion of Innovation*. New York: Free Press.

Valente, Thomas. (1995). *Network Models of the Diffusion of Innovations*. Cresskill, NJ.: Hampton Press.

Watkins, Susan C.. (1991). More lessons from the past: women's informal networks and fertility decline. Paper presented at the IUSSP seminar on Fertility in Subs-Saharan Africa, Harare, Zimbabwe, November 1991.

3

SOCIAL IDENTITY AND COMMUNITY IN THE FERTILITY OF SOUTHERN ETHIOPIAN WOMEN

Dennis P. Hogan and Betemariam Berhanu

INTRODUCTION

This research grows out of a long line of research on ethnic differences in fertility in developed and developing countries. Especially at issue is whether ethnic groups that are in the minority maintain higher-than-expected fertility given their patterns of residence and sociodemographic characteristics. In many developing nations, the focus has been less on diversity in ethnic identity than on the way in which particular traditional religious or ethnic cultural beliefs and practices affect the role of women and reproduction. This research is unique in its focus on a nation, Ethiopia, that is synonymous with ethnic, linguistic, and religious diversity. No group is ascendant in all areas of the nation; the ethnic groups are mixed residentially in some communities and are segregated in others. While all observers agree that the unique personal identities that result from this diversity are fundamental elements of social organization, attitudes, and behaviors, there has been no systematic treatment of these issues. This is in some part due to the political sensitivity of such studies and their potential results.

As in many African counties, ethnic groups in Ethiopia have remained quite distinct for a long period. This long period of exclusiveness, compounded by ethnic competition for political power, resulted in increased intensity of ethnic affiliation. Ethnic commitments in Ethiopia intensified after the new government came to power in May 1991. Since then an increasing number of ethnic-based political parties have been formed and new federal regions have been demarcated along ethnic lines. This in turn has led to a greater ethnic sentiment and increasing variety in its social institutions, and the issue of numerical strength has gained salience, especially among minority ethnic groups. Given this increasing pattern of ethnic intensity, any differences in fertility and fertility-related behaviors will have important social, economic, and political consequences for the future of the nation.

This research is designed to overcome gaps in the social science research understanding of social identity and its relationships to population dynamics. This will be accomplished through the following analytic goals:

1. Measure personal and couple identification of ethnic and religious identity and how these jointly define ethnoreligious group identity;
2. Determine the extent to which these aspects of social identity distinguish key groups in the population, in diverse and homogeneous local communities; and
3. Determine the effects of social identity and community group membership on reproductive behaviors, influencing the demographic dynamics of places and groups within the society.

This chapter is organized into six sections. The next section provides a short description of the Southern Nations, Nationalities, and People's Region (SNNPR). Section three is a brief review of previous studies on ethnic and religious fertility differentials and discusses the applicability of their hypotheses in the Ethiopian context. In section four, we present our data source and operational definitions of variables, and discuss data quality and methods of analysis. Section five presents the findings of the study in three subsections. The first subsection describes the sample population; the second explores ethnic and religious identities of women in the sample and their husbands; and the third investigates ethnoreligious variations in fertility and marital behaviors. Finally, in section six, we summarize the main findings of the study, make conclusions, and provide some policy recommendations.

THE SETTING

The SNNPR is one of the ten federal regions of Ethiopia (see Fig. 3.1). It has a land area of 117,506 square kilometers and a population of 11.1 million in mid-1997 (Table 3.1). Made up of poor farming villages, the region accounts for over one-tenth of Ethiopia's land area, and about one-fifth of its national population. Although the SNNPR has the highest population density in the country with 95 persons per square kilometer, it is one of the least urbanized regions of Ethiopia (Table 3.1). In 1997, less than 7 percent of its population was living in urban areas; the largest city is Awassa, the regional capital, with a population of 69,000. This densely populated region is also characterized by high infant and child mortality, a high level of fertility, and an extremely low level of contraceptive use. As of 1997, the region exhibits an infant mortality rate (IMR) of 102 deaths for every 1,000 live births, and a total fertility rate (TFR) of 6.8 children per woman (Table 3.1).

Fig. 3.1
Map of Ethiopia and the Study Area

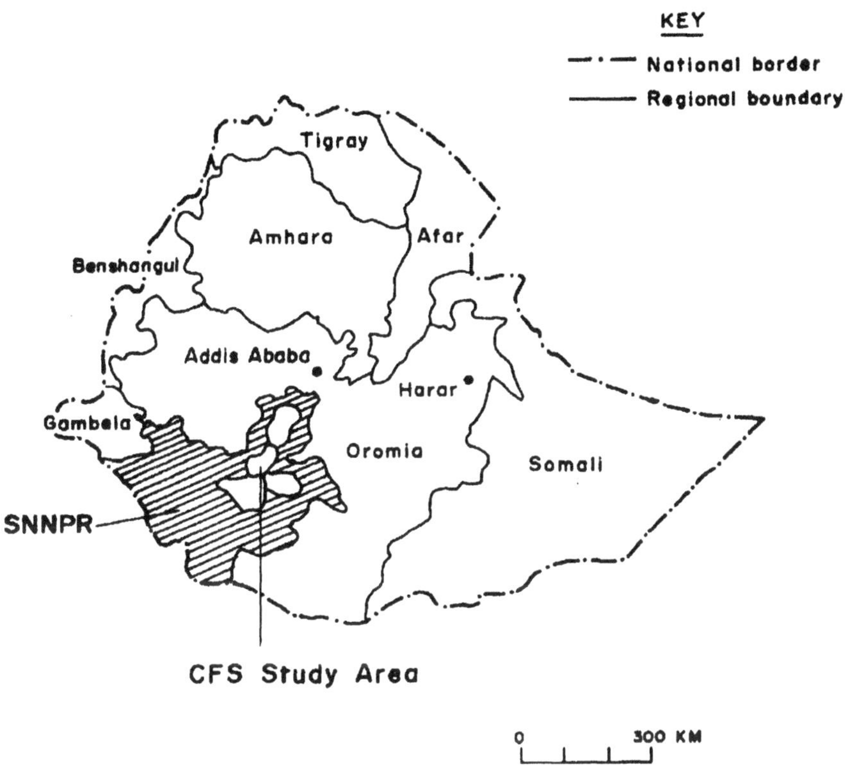

The SNNPR is an extremely ethnically diverse region of Ethiopia, inhabited by more than 80 ethnic groups, of which over 45 (or 56 percent) are indigenous to the region (CSA 1996). These ethnic groups are distinguished by different languages, cultures, and socioeconomic organizations. Although none of the indigenous ethnic groups dominates the ethnic makeup of the national population, there is a considerable ethnic imbalance within the region. The largest ethnic groups in the SNNPR are the Sidama (17.6 percent), Wolayta (11.7 percent), Gurage (8.8 percent), Hadiya (8.4 percent), Selite (7.1 percent), Gamo (6.7 percent), Keffa (5.3 percent), Gedeo (4.4 percent), and Kembata (4.3 percent) (Table 3.1). While the Sidama are the largest ethnic group in the region, each ethnic group is numerically dominant in its respective administrative zone, and there are large minority ethnic groups in each zone. The languages spoken in the SNNPR can be classified into four linguistic families: Cushitic, Nilotic, Omotic, and Semitic. The majority of the ethnic groups in the region are from the family of Omotic language, and ethnic groups belonging to the Nilotic language family are mostly minority. Among the largest ethnic groups, the Gamo, Goffa, and Wolayta are members of the Omotic linguistic family. While the

Hadiya, Kembata, and Sidama are from the Cushitic linguistic group, the Gurage and Amhara belong to the Semitic language family (BOPED 1996).

Table 3.1
Geodemographic Profile of the SNNPR, 1997

Characteristics	
Population Dynamics[1]	
Population Size (million)	11.1
Land Area (sq. kilometers)	117,506
Population density (per sq. km)	95
Urban population (%)	6.7
TFR (per woman)	6.8
IMR (per 1000 live births)	102
Ethnic and Religious Composition [2]	
Ethnic Groups	Percent
Sidama	17.55
Wolayta	11.67
Gurage	8.80
Hadiya	8.43
Selite	7.09
Gamo	6.73
Kefa	5.32
Gedeo	4.43
Kembata	4.28
Amhara	3.01
Kullo	2.63
Goffa	2.32
Oromo	1.99
Bench	1.66
Ari	1.49
Konso	1.36
Alaba	1.13
Koyra	1.01
Timbaro	0.82
Others	8.28
Total	100.00
Religious Groups	
Protestants	34.83
Orthodox Christians	27.60
Moslems	16.73
Traditional	15.37
Catholics	2.97
Others	2.50
Total	100.00

Sources: (1) DTRC/PSTC (1998). (2) CSA (1996), pp. 52–53 and 65.

The SNNPR is also diverse in terms of its religious composition, and differs from other regions due to its experience with strong Protestant missionary activity. There are five major religions: Orthodox Christianity, Roman Catholicism, Protestantism, Islam, and Traditional (non-monotheistic). Protestants form the largest religious group, accounting for about 35 percent of the population. Orthodox Christians and Moslems constitute the second and third largest religious groups in the region, comprising 28 and 17 percent of its population, respectively (Table 3.1). Over 15 percent of the population of the SNNPR adheres to traditional beliefs or has no religion. Other religions (Behais, Jehovahs, Jews, etc.) are but an insignificant minority, barely 2.5 percent (Table 3.1).

The extreme ethnic, religious, and linguistic diversity of the population makes the SNNPR an ideal setting in which to explore ethnic and religious identities of individuals, and how these sources of identity influence fertility behavior. The various ethnic and religious groups intersect and differ in a variety of ways, producing distinctive patterns of individual identity. Some communities are relatively homogeneous with others being quite diverse. It is a fundamental belief of nearly all providers of reproductive health services and most researchers that this extreme level of heterogeneity produces uniquely diverse cultures in which there are great difficulties in promoting fertility limitation and contraceptive use. Ethnographic community studies are better suited to the description of commonalties rather than diversity within communities and rarely provide information on heterogeneity among villages. Demographic microsurvey data on individuals in multiple communities are well suited to addressing the question of the influence of identity and community on reproductive outcomes.

This study of social identity and fertility in the SNNPR is useful for the information it can provide about reproductive-related behaviors in a diverse but neglected African population. It also serves as a useful case study, providing insights into the new patterns of African population dynamics that emerge in multiple crises and characterized by ethnic and religious diversity. The results of this study can also be helpful in the formulation and implementation of population programs that are better suited to the conditions affecting the fertility and contraceptive behavior of different ethnoreligious groups.

PREVIOUS RESEARCH

The roles of ethnicity and religion as determinants of fertility have been the subject of considerable discussion in the fertility literature in both developed and developing countries. Although no consensus has been reached on the mechanisms through which ethnicity and religion affect fertility, three major explanations dominate the literature. These are the assimilation (or characteristics) hypothesis, minority-group status hypothesis, and cultural hypothesis (Goldscheider and Uhlenberg 1969; Ritchey 1975; Jiobu and Marshall 1977; Mosher and Hendershot 1984; Mosher and Goldscheider 1984; Mosher et al. 1986; Stephen et al. 1988; Kollehlon 1989; Pick et al. 1989; Forste and Tienda 1996).

The first explanation, the assimilation hypothesis, suggests that differences in reproductive outcomes between majority and minority ethnic or religious groups are due to differences in socioeconomic and demographic factors. To put it simply, the effect of ethnic or religious group membership is spurious (because ethnic/religious group membership is correlated with socioeconomic and demographic factors known to affect reproductive behavior) or indirect (because membership in an ethnic/religious group may affect the socioeconomic and demographic factors). This suggests that once compositional differences are controlled, differentials in fertility outcomes will disappear.

The second hypothesis, the minority-group status hypothesis, admits the relevance of socioeconomic and demographic factors in explaining differences in reproductive-related outcomes between the majority and minority groups, but asserts that minority-group status exerts an independent influence on fertility behavior. This hypothesis states that the fertility of the minority group will be lower (or the use of contraceptives will be higher) than that of the majority group if certain conditions are met. These conditions include: the minority group must have similar socioeconomic and demographic attributes as the majority group; the group must not have pronatalist norms, instead desiring to acculturate the values of the majority group; and the minority group must have aspirations for upward mobility with no feelings of insecurity and marginality. When these conditions are not met, the minority group will have higher fertility (or lower contraceptive use) than the majority group.

The third explanation, the cultural hypothesis, postulates that ethnic/religious group differentials in reproductive-related behavior may be due to differences in norms, values, and attitudes toward fertility-related behavior among ethnic/religious groups. Distinctive aspects of cultures or norms about fertility and fertility control may produce distinct patterns of fertility outcomes among different ethnic/religious groups. Hill (1985), in his study in Mali, also noted that the very different lifestyles of different ethnic groups in many African countries may lead to different patterns of fertility behavior even though they live in comparable physical settings.

One common limitation of the above three hypotheses is the assumption that institutional factors affecting fertility behavior (such as family planning services and government policies) are equally available to, or affect, members of different ethnic/religious groups. Their implicit assumption is that what determines differences in fertility behavior between minority and majority groups is individuals' orientation toward family size and contraceptive use, but not the institutional contexts in which reproductive behavior takes place. To overcome this drawback, recent studies have emphasized the role of community characteristics and government policies in understanding ethnic and religious differentials in fertility (Murty and De Vos 1984; Govindasamy and DaVanzo 1992; Forste and Tienda 1996).

These studies contend that, while minority-group status and socioeconomic and cultural factors undoubtedly play important roles in accounting for ethnic or religious differentials in fertility, such differentials must also be caused by community characteristics and government policies and programs. Murty and

De Vos (1984), for example, argue that ethnic discrimination in the provision of family planning services, or discomfort in discussing sensitive topics such as reproduction with someone outside of one's ethnic group, or language barrier could explain ethnic differences in fertility and contraceptive use. Others attribute ethnic and religious differentials in fertility-related behaviors to varying ethnic/religious groups' responses to broad-based government policies and programs (Govindasamy and DaVanzo 1992). It is argued that ethnocentric practices in developing countries, such as the channeling of scarce public resources to areas where members of dominant elites are concentrated, subsequently creates social inequality by benefiting members of some ethnic groups more than others. This in turn leads to demographic diversity among ethnic and religious groups.

Another limitation of previous studies of ethnic and religious fertility differentials is that they all consider ethnicity and religion as two distinct attributes. We shall show later that neither ethnicity nor religion by itself is an adequate specification of an individual's social identity and shall therefore consider the relevance of ethnic differences within religious groups. The third, but most important, limitation of previous demographic research is the little emphasis given to community ethnic or religious diversity in understanding ethnic/religious fertility differentials. We argue that, drawing upon the sociological tradition, human reproduction occurs in and is influenced by a social context in which diversity is an important element. While family-planning services and other structural community characteristics are important, community diversity may also manifest itself as a variety of potential effects that shape reproductive behaviors. For example, as is often the case in many African countries, diversity brings a very difficult problem of social identity. Each identity group may feel that its safety lies in its size and proportion. This anxiety over numbers is an obstacle for efforts to reduce fertility levels or increase the provision of family planning services (Pai Panandiker and Umashankar 1994).

In addition, demographic studies of innovation and diffusion have shown that communities serve as social networks through which information and new ideas flow (Bongaarts and Watkins 1996; Montgomery and Casterline 1996). These studies further indicated that characteristics of networks are relevant for the diffusion of new ideas and information about smaller family size and contraceptive use. Research in Kenya, for example, has revealed that personal networks in which fertility preferences and family planning were discussed were relatively homogeneous (Bongaarts and Watkins 1996). In the United States, in contrast, Granovetter (1974) found that information about job opportunities was less readily available in socially homogeneous groups than in heterogeneous groups. Similarly, Bott (1971) indicated that homogeneous networks permitted less autonomy for innovative behavior with regard to the division of household labor by gender. Extending these ideas to fertility change, one can argue that, depending on socioeconomic and cultural contexts, community diversity may either inhibit fertility change, or serve to promote the diffusion of new ideas and information about fertility limitation and contraception. While we cannot a priori predict the direction of the probable effects, we expect community diversity to have important influences on the fertility and fertility-related behaviors of women in the SNNPR.

We consider the usefulness of the assimilation, minority-group status, and norms hypotheses for understanding the patterns of reproductive-related behaviors within the SNNPR context. We also consider the role of community diversity and service availability, as well that of marital homogamy, in explaining the fertility behavior of women in the SNNPR. We ask whether different ethnoreligious groups, majority and minority groups, endogamous and exogamous women, and diverse and homogeneous communities are likely to have different patterns of reproductive behaviors. We believe, however, that testing the minority-group status hypothesis with the type of data we have, and within the socioeconomic context of the SNNPR, is difficult. We use this hypothesis as a theoretical guide to examine whether membership in a dominant group in a local community has any impact on the reproductive behavior of women.

DATA AND METHODS

The Data

The data used in this study come from the Community and Family Survey (CFS) conducted in May 1997. The CFS, a regional representative survey covering SNNPR, was a collaborative project of the Demographic Training and Research Center (DTRC) of Addis Ababa University and the Population Studies and Training Center (PSTC) of Brown University (DTRC/PSTC 1998).

The CFS was a stratified probability sample of women aged 15–49. Households were identified using a three-stage cluster sampling procedure. Five major zones in the region were first selected. These zones represent about 80 percent of the population of the SNNPR. (The remaining 20 percent live in extremely remote mountainous and lowland areas) (see Fig. 3.1).

The five selected zones were stratified into rural and urban areas. In the rural stratum, one highland and one lowland *wereda* (a unit roughly similar to a New England township) were selected at random from each zone to capture agricultural ecology niches. The urban sample is representative of the selected zones as a whole. Twenty-nine communities (20 rural villages and 9 urban centers) were selected at random for the survey. All eligible women in the selected households were successfully interviewed, resulting in a final sample of 2,550 women aged 15–49 (DTRC/PSTC 1998).

This 1997 microlevel survey gathered a wealth of information on the marital and fertility behaviors of women aged 15–49, and on their family and community situations. Information was also collected on the household situation (from heads of households), and the community (from knowledgeable community leaders). In this chapter, we use data for 1,375 currently married women in their first marriage who are ages 20–49 and married to the household head. We include women who are ages 20 and older because of selection biases on marriage for younger women. Marriage and reproductive outcomes were collected from the individual respondent. Information on the ethnic origin, religion, and religious devotion of these women and their husbands was obtained from the household record as reported by the household head.

An assessment of the data collected in the 1997 CFS showed that the data are of good quality. The response rate for household interviews was 95 percent; for individual interviews it was almost 100 percent (DTRC/PSTC 1998). Previous analysis of information collected in the 1997 CFS also revealed no serious biases, misreporting, missing cases, or out-of-range values (Hogan et. al. 1999).

MEASURING ETHNIC AND RELIGIOUS IDENTITIES

Ethnic Identity. The ethnic identity of the respondent and her husband was determined from the response of the household head to the following question: "To what ethnic group does [name] belong?" Although the CFS identified 52 ethnic groups in the study area, we consider only eight major ethnic groups (Amhara, Gurage, Hadiya, Kembata/Timbaro, Konta, Selite, Sidama, and Wolayta) and the remaining were lumped together to form "Other" ethnic groups. This was done to maintain a reasonable number of women in each ethnic category. The Kemabata and Timbaro each formed a very small percentage in the sample, and hence we decided to group them in one ethnic category because they are culturally similar and adjacent.

Mother Tongue. The CFS asked each ever-married woman whether she and her first husband had the same mother tongue (language) before they got married. If the answer was no, then she was further asked whose language she and her husband speak in their home.

Religious Identity. The religious identity of the respondent and her husband was determined from the response of the household head report to the question "What is [name's] religious denomination?" The responses to this question were divided into six religious groups: (1) Orthodox Christian, (2) Catholic, (3) Protestant, (4) Moslem, (5) Traditional (i.e., persons without religious identification or those who adhere to traditional beliefs), and (6) Others (Behais, Johovas, Jews, etc). The CFS also asked each ever-married woman whether she and her first husband had the same religion before they got married. If the answer was no, then she was further asked whose religion she practiced after marrying her first husband. We use this information to determine whether the respondent and her husband had different religions before her marriage.

Ethnoreligious Identity. We use ethnic and religious identities of women and their husbands to identify their ethnoreligious groups. Theoretically, there are 54 (9 x 6) possible combinations of ethnic and religious identities. However, to maintain a reasonable number of cases (at least 30 women) in each cell, we consider only 22 distinct, but bounded, ethnoreligious groups. Most of our discussions and interpretations of the results apply to these ethnoreligious groups.

Religious Devotion. Devotionalism was measured from the reports of the household head to a series of questions on religious practices of each household member. These questions were different for Christians, Moslems, and Traditionals. Christians were asked how often they attend church services, say their prayers, and observe fasting. Moslems and Traditionals[1] were asked how often they say their prayers and observe their fasting periods. The responses to these questions were grouped into "often," "sometime," and "never." Respondents who answered "often" for each of these questions were considered *highly devotional.*

Ethnoreligious Majority Status in a Community. We defined a respondent woman as "ethnic majority," "religious majority," or "ethnoreligious majority" if her ethnic, religious, or ethnoreligious identity is the most common in her community. In this study, "community" is defined as *kebele,* the smallest administrative unit in Ethiopia: the peasants' association (PA) in rural areas and the urban dwellers' association (UDA) in urban areas. As noted above, the CFS covered 29 kebeles (20 PAs and 9 UDAs) (DTRC/PSTC 1998).

COMMUNITY MEASURES

We use three measures to explore the effects of community on fertility behavior of women. We identify whether a community is rural or urban. We also include a measure of availability of contraceptive services in a community to capture the effects of family planning information or education and methods on fertility outcomes. Our principal community measure is, however, ethnoreligious diversity. We determine whether a community is "homogeneous" or "diverse" using a measure of diversity called the "entropy index" (White 1986).

The entropy index is defined as:

$$H_i = - \sum_{k=1}^{K} P_{ik} \ln(P_{ik})$$

where $i = 1$ to I (I = 29 is number of communities).

$P_{ik} = N_{ik} / N_i$

N_{ik}= number of persons in k^{th} ethnic or religious group in the ith community,

N_i = total population size of the ith community, and

K = total number of ethnic, religious, or ethnoreligious groups in the SNNPR.

The entropy index is not bounded from above. Since comparison is our main interest here, we normed this index by dividing by its maximum value, ln(K), where K is as defined above. The resulting index has a value that ranges between 0 and 1. Larger values of this index (close to 1) indicate ethnic or religious diversity in a community, whereas lower values of the index (close to 0) suggest homogeneity in ethnoreligious composition. To facilitate interpretations of results, we divide communities into three groups: diverse, intermediate, and homogeneous. Communities whose index values fall in the top and lower 25 percent of the distribution are considered as diverse and homogeneous, respectively. Those whose values fall in the middle 50 percent of the distribution are referred to as intermediate. For the purpose of multivariate analyses, we recode this variable into an ordinal scale as 0 = homogeneous, 1 = intermediate, and 2 = diverse.

The use of community variables in the models means that the data include multiple women from the same *kebele*, and therefore that the observations are not independent. We have corrected this problem by adjusting the standard errors of the estimated coefficients for clustering effects using the Huber correction procedure in Stata (StataCorp 1999). Because we restrict the analysis to currently married women aged 20–49 who were in their first marriage and married to the household head, our study includes only one eligible woman from each household; consequently there is no problem of intrahousehold correlation.

MEASURING OUTCOMES

In this chapter, we examine the fertility and marital behavior of women in the SNNPR using six common measures of reproductive behavior. We use *children ever born and recent fertility*, *lifetime fertility intentions*, and *current or future contraceptive use* to measure actual fertility and fertility preferences of women. We explore ethnoreligious differences in the timing and patterns of marriage using *age at first marriage, the age difference between spouses*, and *marriage to a husband with more than one wife*. These measures are selected based on their theoretical and empirical significance. Demographic research has clearly demonstrated that marriage is the principal determinant of fertility exposure in developing countries. Both the timing of first marriage and the age difference between spouses are important factors affecting the timing of childbearing, completed family size, fertility preferences, and contraceptive use. The age difference between spouses also influences the position of women in a society, a factor that has a direct bearing on fertility (Casterline et al. 1986; Hogan et al. 1999). The significance of the institution of polygyny for fertility and contraceptive use has also been shown by many studies. Polygyny is often associated with women's low status and gender inequality within marriage, which in turn translates into high fertility patterns and low level of contraceptive use (Boye et al. 1991; Ezeh 1997).

The age difference between spouses is calculated as the difference in years between the husband's age and that of the wife at the time of the survey.

Children ever born is obtained from information in which the woman indicates the numbers of sons and daughters ever born. We measure recent fertility of the women using information on the number of children born to them between 1991 and 1997. By controlling for the number of children alive in 1990, this analysis of recent fertility is similar to a parity progression study and is conditioned on the number of children already born.

Lifetime fertility intentions are measured from the response to the question on the ideal number of children that a respondent would want to have in her life. This variable was grouped into two categories: those who believe that the number of children is up to God or those who said they do not know, and those who reported some number.

Current or Future Use of Contraceptives. Contraceptive prevalence rate is extremely low in the study area. Women interviewed in the CFS were asked: "Do you or your husband currently use any family planning method to avoid or delay getting pregnant?" In response, only 2 percent of currently married women aged 15–49 answered yes (Hogan et al. 1999). Those not using a method were then asked: "Do you or your husband intend to use any family planning methods in the future?" About one-fifth of the women responded affirmatively, indicating a predisposition toward future use. In Ethiopia, where use of modern contraceptive methods has just begun, we expect that effects of ethnoreligious group membership and community diversity on contraception are more likely to be expressed in receptivity toward future use rather than in use per se. Using this information, we construct a binary dependent variable "Contraceptive Use/ Plan." This variable is coded as 1 if the respondent is *currently using or intends to use in the future*, and 0 if she is not currently using or intending to use in the future.

In modeling all these outcomes, we control for a number of confounding factors that have theoretical significance and are available in our data set.[2]

Methods of Analysis

The analysis in this study uses both descriptive and multivariate techniques.[3] The multivariate methods we employ depend on the nature of the dependent variable. We use OLS (Ordinary Least Squares) regression methods to model the age at first marriage and age difference between spouses. To model whether lifetime fertility is seen as "up to God" and current or future contraceptive adoption, we estimate logistic regression models. In modeling children ever born and recent fertility, we employ poisson regression models for count data (Agresti 1996). The results of the estimated poisson regression models are incidence rate ratios (relative risk ratios). An incidence ratio of 1.00 indicates that the independent variable has no effect. An incidence ratio greater than 1.00 indicates an increased likelihood of a given outcome relative to the likelihood of being in the reference category. An incidence ratio less than 1.00 indicates a reduced likelihood of a given outcome relative to the likelihood of being in the reference group.

FINDINGS

Description of the Sample Population

The SNNPR is a poor, uneducated population at a very early stage of the fertility and mortality transitions (Table 3.2). Less than 10 percent of women and only one-quarter of husbands are literate. More than 95 percent of these women were born and live in a rural community. Age at marriage is under age 15 for about one-fifth of all women, with more women marrying at ages 15–19. A majority of women marry men from the same village or town. Forty-one percent of the women have husbands who are ten or more years older. More than one-quarter of the women are in marriages in which the husband has at least one additional wife. The mean number of children ever born is 4.2, and more than one-third of the women have experienced one or more child deaths.

There is little recognition of fertility limitation, with almost two-thirds of women unable to name an ideal number of children they want to have, responding instead that their lifetime family size is "up to God." Over one-half wanted another child soon, with most of the remainder desiring to space rather than limit their births. Only one-third of the women have access to family planning services from any source. Consistent with this, only 37 percent of women know at least one method of family planning, and only 4 percent of these currently married women were using a family planning method at the time of the study. However, there seems to be some interest in contraceptive use over the lifetime; over one-fifth of the respondents indicated their intention to use family planning methods sometime in the future.

The values of the entropy index suggest that although the SNNPR as a whole is extremely diverse in terms of ethnic and religious composition of its population, ethnic and religious groups live mostly in very homogeneous communities (*kebeles*) (Table 3.2). This is particularly true for ethnic groups where the value of the entropy index is very small (less than 11 percent). A further look at this index decomposed by rural and urban communities (not shown here) reveals that rural *kebeles* are more homogeneous than urban *kebeles*, a fact that may be attributed to rural-urban migration.

Table 3.2
Sociodemographic Characteristics of the Study Women, Currently Married Women in First Marriage Ages 20–49: Southern Ethiopia, 1997

Variables	%[a]	Variables	%[a]
Age		Ideal Number of Children	
20–29	48.3	1–3	0.8
30–39	34.9	4–6	21.8
40–49	16.7	7 or more	13.6
Mean (years)	30.7	"Up to God" /Don't Know	63.8

Continued

Variables	%[a]	Variables	%[a]
Age at First Marriage		Fertility Desire	
10–14	20.3	Want to Limit	11.2
15–19	33.6	Want to Space	34.5
20 or older	22.1	Want More Soon	54.3
Mean (years)	17.0		
		Contraceptive Behavior	
Duration of Marriage		Knowledge of Any Method	37.2
<10 years	13.7	Current Use	3.6
10–19	35.6	Intend to Use in Future	20.2
20 or more years	36.1	Husband-wife family planning communication	29.2
Mean (years)	28.3		
Husband-wife Age Difference		Socioeconomic Factors	
< 10	58.7	Literate	9.6
10–19	33.1	Husband Literate	24.7
20 or more	8.1		
Mean (years)	9.3	Community Factors	
		Community Diversity[a]	
Polygynous Marriage	28.6	Ethnic Composition (mean/100)	10.4
Number of Children Ever born		Religious Composition	33.3
0	6.2	Ethnoreligious Composition	17.6
1–3	41.2	Rural Place of Birth	96.4
4–6	29.9	Rural Residence	95.0
7 or more	22.7	Husband/Wife Lived in Same Village/town before Marriage	55.1
Mean (number)	4.2		
% With 1 + Child Death	36.1		
		Community Family Planning Service	32.0
Mean (number)	0.8		
		Number of Women	1375

Notes: Percentages are weighted and may not add to 100 because of rounding. N (Number of cases) is unweighted.
[a] Means (per 100) of the Entropy Index.

Ethnic and Religious Identities and Marital Homogamy

The diversity of membership in the major ethnic groups in the SNNPR is displayed in Table 3.3. The ethnic groups vary remarkably in size, from fewer than 2 percent who are Amhara to more than one-fifth who are Konta or Sidama. Overall, 92 percent of women "self-select" (that is, they marry either because of their own choice or under the influence of their family) a man from the same ethnic group. For those few groups who are combinations of smaller ethnic groups and seem to depart from this pattern, a high degree of marital homogamy is evident in the proclivity of women to marry men with the same mother tongue. Except for the smallest Amhara and mixed groups, most women live in communities in which their ethnic group is dominant.

Table 3.3
Percent Distribution of Respondents and Husbands by Ethnic Identity, Self-selection, Dominance, and Religious Devotion, Currently Married Women in First Marriage Ages 20–49: Southern Ethiopia, 1997

Ethnic Group	% Women	% Husbands	% Self-selection: Ethnic group	% Self-selection: Mother tongue	% Ethnic Majority	% Religiously Devoted
Amhara	1.4	1.0	32.6	71.5	15.5	63.5
Gurage	6.6	6.8	96.6	96.3	84.4	48.1
Hadiya	13.4	12.5	80.8	96.1	81.9	59.6
Kembata/Timbaro	4.1	4.4	53.9	82.8	61.7	52.8
Konta	20.7	20.8	100.0	98.4	100.0	0.4
Sidama	25.9	26.0	99.5	99.9	99.3	41.9
Selite	13.7	13.6	98.4	95.7	98.8	20.1
Wolayta	8.6	8.6	96.7	98.6	94.1	47.0
Others	5.5	6.3	67.2	91.5	27.0	55.4
Total	100.0	100.0	91.9	96.6	88.9	35.0
N (unweighted)	1375	1375				

Note: Percentages are weighted and may not add to 100 because of rounding.

Table 3.4
Percent Distribution of Women and Husbands by Religious Identity, Self-selection, Dominance, and Religious Devotion, Currently Married Women in First Marriage Ages 20–49: Southern Ethiopia, 1997

Religious Group	% Women	% Husbands	% Self-selection	% Religiously Devoted	% Religious Majority
Orthodox	24.2	24.4	96.4	26.1	53.9
Catholic	3.6	3.6	88.3	16.8	0.0
Protestant	32.2	31.1	90.3	61.0	90.9
Moslem	19.7	19.7	93.0	33.8	88.6
Traditional	17.0	18.0	85.9	0.0	67.4
Others	3.3	3.3	97.6	54.0	0.0
Total	100.0	100.0	91.7	35.0	71.2
N	1375	1375			

Notes: Percentages are weighted and may not add to 100 because of rounding. Number of women (N) is unweighted. Index of dissimilarity between marriage and current religious distribution is 24.2.

A similar analysis of homogamy in religious sect is provided in Table 3.4. In the SNNPR Protestant missionaries have made substantial inroads into the population, converting one-third of the residents. The Christian Orthodox and Moslem religions are the other major sects. Religious homogamy in marriage is as strong as ethnic homogamy, with 92 percent of the women marrying husbands who are of the same religion. The Christian Orthodox often express concern about retaining its members from one generation to the next. These data suggest that, at least in the South of Ethiopia, they have had remarkable success with fewer than 4 percent of Christian Orthodox religion marrying a person from another religion. However, smaller proportions of the Christian Orthodox report high religious devotion, with Protestants (61 percent) especially displaying considerable devotional commitment. Protestant and Moslem women tend to live in communities in which they are the majority; only one-half of the Orthodox live in communities in which the Orthodox dominate.

Table 3.5
Percent Distribution of Women and Husbands by Ethnoreligious Group Membership, Self-selection, Group Dominance, and Religious Devotion, Currently Married Women in First Marriage Ages 20–49: Southern Ethiopia, 1997

Ethnoreligious Groups	% Women	% Husbands	% Self-selection: Ethno-religion	% Self-selection: Ethno-Religion & Language	% Religiously Devoted	% Ethno-Religious Majority
Orthodox Christians						
1. Amhara	1.1	0.8	39.8	35.4	58.4	4.4
2. Gurage	5.3	5.4	98.4	98.4	50.2	94.9
3. Hadiya	2.4	2.2	65.0	60.6	24.7	3.4
4. Kembata/ Timbaro	1.1	0.9	44.2	32.5	17.7	0.0
5. Konta	8.1	8.1	100.0	95.9	1.1	46.6
6. Wolayta	3.9	4.0	94.7	94.7	35.2	69.4
7. Other ethnic group	2.1	2.9	81.1	79.1	36.5	1.0
Catholics and Other Christians						
8. Kembata/ Timbaro	0.8	0.8	97.9	71.8	5.8	0.0
9. Sidama	4.6	4.5	96.9	96.9	34.6	0.0
10. Other ethnic group	1.4	1.5	88.8	88.8	39.5	0.0
Protestant Christians						
11. Hadiya	7.0	6.8	76.4	75.4	76.8	65.6
12. Kembata/ Timbaro	2.2	2.1	55.1	51.2	84.9	71.5
13. Sidama	15.9	15.2	94.2	94.2	46.5	98.6
14. Wolayta	4.1	4.1	92.6	92.6	63.5	69.4
15. Other ethnic group	2.9	2.8	44.7	44.7	81.1	39.9

Continued

Ethnoreligious Groups	% Women	% Husbands	% Self-selection Ethno-religion	Ethno-Religion & Language	% Religiously Devoted	% Ethno-Religious Majority
Moslems						
16. Gurage	1.0	1.2	92.6	82.4	40.6	26.5
17. Hadiya	2.6	2.7	94.9	94.0	60.1	97.6
18. Selite	13.7	13.6	98.4	94.5	20.1	98.8
19. Other ethnic group	2.5	2.2	84.4	83.5	80.3	88.1
Traditional						
20. Konta	12.3	12.3	100.0	100.0	0.0	0.0
21. Sidama	3.0	3.8	97.2	97.2	0.0	0.0
22. Other ethnic group	1.8	1.9	67.0	67.0	0.0	0.0
Total	100.0	100.0	90.0	88.4	35.0	64.8
N	1375	1375				

Note: Percentages are weighted and may not add to 100 because rounding.

After extensive experimentation, comparing indices of dissimilarities and other measures of the social distances of groups and in light of the number of sample cases available, we identified twenty-two ethnoreligious groups (that is, groups defined by both ethnicity and religion of the women) (Table 3.5) for further examination. The strongest evidence of the appropriateness of these combined groups as social identities is the persistently high degree of marital homogamy (90 percent) observed in these much more refined groups. This is remarkable given the increased number of groups and the much smaller proportions of each of the groups in the population. While the level of homogamy tended to be smaller for groups that were not majorities in their communities, the relationship was by no means perfect (e.g., Catholics/Other Christians in Sidama and Kembata/Timbaro had a 97 percent rate of self-selection, even though almost all of that population lived in communities in which they were not the dominant group). The utility of these twenty-two ethnoreligious groups for analysis is demonstrated by the tremendous diversity in the degree of homogamy among ethnic groups within religious groupings. There is little advantage to adding language to this definition of ethnoreligious groups, since these seem to capture all relevant aspects of social identity.

Table 3.6
Fertility and Marital Behavior of Respondents, by Ethnoreligious Group Membership, Spousal Selection, and Community Diversity, Currently Married Women in First Marriage Ages 20–49 (N = 1375): Southern Ethiopia, 1997

	Mean			Percentage		
	Age at First Marriage	Spousal Age Difference	NCEB	Polygynous Union	Ideal Family Size "Up To God"	Family Planning Use/ Plan
Ethnoreligious Groups	*	*	*	*	*	*
Orthodox Christians						
Amhara	17.5	8.4	3.8	4.4	40.9	59.3
Gurage	15.8	11.1	4.8	23.7	95.9	3.2
Hadiya	18.8	10.8	6.4	29.2	76.0	23.5
Kembata/Timbaro	18.8	8.4	5.1	40.6	44.6	45.2
Konta	16.3	9.2	3.8	26.7	52.1	31.5
Wolayta	19.4	9.6	4.9	19.9	46.3	46.5
Other ethnic group	18.0	8.0	4.7	3.9	44.7	25.9
Catholics and Other Christians						
Kembata/Timbaro	21.1	12.1	3.0	26.1	95.7	2.1
Sidama	14.1	9.7	4.3	36.9	50.8	23.9
Other ethnic group	19.3	8.0	4.9	40.8	75.3	25.0
Protestant Christians						
Hadiya	18.7	7.3	4.5	26.1	77.6	22.1
Kembata/Timbaro	19.0	8.5	4.3	17.0	63.3	23.2
Sidama	15.7	10.7	4.4	36.9	43.6	26.7
Wolayta	20.3	6.6	3.5	15.5	50.7	57.0
Other ethnic group	18.5	6.7	4.0	9.3	35.6	36.1
Moslems						
Gurage	16.5	13.5	3.8	33.7	85.8	5.4
Hadiya	19.9	9.3	4.5	27.3	53.9	4.5
Selite	16.6	9.0	4.3	41.1	95.7	0.6
Other ethnic group	14.9	13.3	5.6	34.6	50.7	5.4
Traditional						
Konta	17.1	7.4	2.7	22.5	66.2	35.5
Sidama	14.6	14.3	5.4	19.1	71.1	13.8
Other ethnic group	15.7	9.9	3.6	34.1	62.4	30.8
Spousal Selection	*	*		*	*	*
Homogamy	16.7	9.5	4.3	29.1	64.7	21.9
Intermarriage	18.2	8.4	4.1	25.8	59.3	33.2
Ethnoreligious Group Status	*	*	*	*	*	*
Majority	17.1	9.1	4.0	29.8	67.4	22.3
Minority	16.8	9.7	4.6	26.3	57.3	26.5
Community Diversity	*	*	*	*	*	*
Homogeneous	16.1	10.5	4.0	38.5	88.9	5.2
Intermediate	17.1	9.0	4.3	27.9	59.1	26.7
Diverse	18.3	8.2	4.6	11.8	38.8	45.4
All Women	***17.0***	***9.3***	***4.2***	***28.6***	***63.8***	***23.8***

Notes: * $p \leq 0.05$. NCEB = Number of Children Ever Born.

Ethnoreligious Variations in Marital and Fertility Behaviors

Age at first marriage varies remarkably across the ethnic groups within religious groups (Table 3.6). For example, among the Orthodox Christians the mean age at marriage is 18.8 or higher for the Hadiya, Kembata/Timbaro, and Wolayta. It is 15.8 among the Gurage. Nor do all Moslems have an early age at marriage, with the Hadiya Moslem women marrying at a mean age of 19.9. Many women are married to husbands who have more than one wife. With the exception of the Orthodox Amhara, this is true of every ethnic group and each religion. More than one-third of women are in this situation among Orthodox Christians who are Kembata/Timbaro, Catholic, or Protestant Sidama, and Moslems who are Gurage or Hadiya.

To summarize major aspects of these variations, we compared mean age at marriage by dimensions of homogamy, community diversity, and ethnoreligious majority status (Table 3.6). Mean marriage age of a woman marrying a man of the same ethnic, religious, and linguistic group is 16.7. A later marriage age of 18.2 is observed among those who differ on one or more dimensions. It might be suspected that this occurs when a young woman fails to find a husband who is fully homogamous, and has to settle for a husband who differs on one of the dimensions of social identity. This argument receives support in the earlier age at marriage of women in homogamous communities where the task of finding a spouse with the same social identity is presumably easier. Being a majority member of the community has a similar impact on age at marriage, although the effect is modest. We estimated a multivariate model of the relationship of being in a homogamous marriage to the timing of marriage, controlling for age cohort, rural origins, and whether the husband and wife are from the same community (Table 3.7). Viewed in this way, there is no relationship between homogamy of the wife and her husband and her age at marriage. Similarly, there is no association between degree of religiosity and the age at first marriage (Table 3.7).

The age difference between spouses varies enormously among the twenty-two ethnoreligious groups, as much as the age at first marriage does. The mean age difference falls short of seven years only among Protestants who belong to the Wolayta and to the smallest mixed ethnic groups (Table 3.6), suggesting preferences for large spousal age differences in the region. This is in conformity to norms about age differences in Southern Ethiopia. The SNNPR, in general, is a society with a custom of the bride joining the household of her husband's family (Hogan et al. 1999). In such a society, there is a strong preference for large spousal age difference since younger wives can be more easily molded into the roles desired by the husband's family (Casterline et al. 1986). The variation among ethnic groups with different religious beliefs is, however, impressive. The mean age difference ranges from 6.6 years among Protestant Wolayta to 14.3 years among Traditional Sidama (Table 3.6). The Gurage observe the highest mean age difference among Orthodox and Protestant Christians, but Protestant Gurage have a higher mean age difference than their Orthodox counterparts. The spousal age difference patterns among the twenty-two ethnoreligious groups observed in Table 3.6, in general, persist with the multivariate controls in Table 3.7.

Table 3.7
Effects of Ethnoreligious Group Membership, Marital Homogamy, and Community Diversity on Age at First Marriage, Spousal Age Difference, and Polygynous Union, Currently Married Women Ages 20–49 (N = 1375): Southern Ethiopia, 1997

	Age at First Marriage	Spousal Age Difference	Polygynous Union
	Parameter Estimate (OLS)		Odds Ratio (Logit)
Ethnoreligious Groups			
Orthodox Christians			
Amhara	1.71*	-1.70*	0.21*
Gurage	0.49	-2.47*	0.43*
Hadiya	2.60*	-2.56*	0.73*
Kembata/Timbaro	3.03*	-0.16	1.08
Konta	0.49	-1.56*	0.84
Wolayta	3.76*	-1.23*	0.80
Other ethnic group	2.88*	-0.95	0.26*
Catholics and Other Christians			
Kembata/Timbaro	4.18*	-1.77*	0.25*
Sidama	-1.33*	0.27	1.13
Other ethnic group	3.57*	-1.09*	1.19
Protestant Christians			
Hadiya	2.94*	-1.31*	0.81*
Kembata/Timbaro	3.60*	-1.68*	0.28*
Sidama	Ref.	Ref.	Ref.
Wolayta	3.53*	-1.28*	0.42*
Other ethnic group	2.97*	-0.70	0.40*
Moslems			
Gurage	2.12*	2.34*	0.81
Hadiya	4.01*	-0.84	0.85
Selite	0.99*	-2.14*	1.14
Other ethnic group	2.81*	-1.23*	0.96
Traditional			
Konta	1.37*	-1.31*	0.96
Sidama	-0.70	0.80	0.76
Other ethnic group	1.23	-2.20*	0.81
Marital Homogamy and Group Status			
Same Ethnic, Religion & Language	-0.26	0.14	0.78
Ethnoreligious Majority	—	0.33	0.90
Religious Devotion	—	-0.84*	0.75*
Community Variables			
Ethnoreligious Diversity	—	-1.18*	0.72*
Urban Place of Birth/ Residence	-0.33	-0.63	0.50*

Continued

	Age at First Marriage	Spousal Age Difference	Polygynous Union
Intercept	15.77*	10.74*	(-0.54)
Model R^2 (%)	23.71	57.52	
Model F-value/Chi-square (df)	19 (27,1347)*	28 (32,1343)*	142(31)*

Notes: OLS models include wife/husband age and literacy, migration status, and spousal age difference. Logistic include age at and duration of marriage. * $p \leq 0.05$.

Comparison of mean age difference by dimensions of homogamy and ethnoreligious majority status reveals only small differences (Table 3.6). These differences disappear when we estimate a multivariate model, controlling for a number of variables (Table 3.7). Thus, as is the case for age at first marriage, there appears to be no relationship between homogamy of the wife and her husband and the age difference between spouses. Nor is there any association between being member of a majority group in the community or degree of religiosity and spousal age difference. In contrast, community diversity appears to be strongly associated with the age difference between spouses (Table 3.7). Other things being equal, women living in homogeneous communities display a significantly larger spousal age difference than women living in diverse communities. This probably has to do with an earlier age at first marriage among women in homogenous communities, as the task of finding a homogamous spouse is relatively easier. It is also possible that norms regarding large age differences between spouses are stronger in homogeneous than heterogeneous communities. Moreover, women living in communities inhabited by diverse ethnoreligious groups may have a relatively higher socioeconomic status. This may mean that such women are less likely to marry early and more likely to find a spouse of approximately the same age (Casterline et al. 1986). These community differences are net of wives' literacy status, but all aspects of women's status is not captured by this single indicator.

Women are more likely to be married to a husband with additional wives in situations in which they are of the same ethnicity, religion, and mother tongue (Table 3.6). Women who live in homogeneous communities and who are in a dominant group in that community are much more often observed in these homogamous marriages. The multivariate model (Table 3.7) confirms that women in communities that are more heterogeneous are less likely to have a husband who has more than one wife, even controlling for urban/rural residence and ethnic group. However, religious dominance in the community does not have an effect. Ethnoreligious groups have distinctive patterns of polygyny taking into account their situations within communities and key characteristics of the women and their marriage. Except for the Orthodox Kembata/Timbaro, women who are Orthodox or Protestant Christians are less likely to have a husband who has an additional wife. It is interesting to note that Kembata/Timbaro women who are Orthodox Christian are more likely to be in polygynous union than their Protestant Christian counterparts (Table 3.7).

There is tremendous ethnic variation within the major religious groups in the proportion of women who believe that the number of children they will have during their lifetime is "up to God." Virtually all of the Orthodox Gurage and three-quarters of the Hadiya have this belief, compared to about one-half of all other Orthodox ethnic groups (Table 3.6). The Gurage and Selite Moslems predominantly hold similar beliefs, but Hadiya Moslems are notably less likely than Orthodox Hadiyas to hold such a view. This belief is common among women in most types of communities, but is especially strong for women in communities that are homogeneous or where their ethnic group is dominant (Table 3.6). This relationship is confirmed in the multivariate model (Table 3.8).

Table 3.8
Effects of Ethnoreligious Group Membership and Status, Marital Homogamy, and Community Diversity on Fertility, Ideal Family Size, and Contraceptive Use/Intention, Currently Married Women in First Marriage Ages 20–49 (N = 1375): Southern Ethiopia, 1997

	No. Children Ever Born		Ideal Family Size "Up to God"	Family Planning Use/Plan
	Total	In 1991–97		
	Relative Risk Ratio (Poisson)		Odds Ratio (Logit)	
Ethnoreligious Groups				
Orthodox Christians				
Amhara	0.83*	0.57*	3.64*	1.15
Gurage	0.95	0.75*	5.91*	0.32*
Hadiya	1.13*	0.89	7.45*	0.54*
Kembata/Timbaro	1.14*	1.02	4.32*	1.21
Konta	0.79*	0.72*	1.23	3.12*
Wolayta	1.05	0.91	3.33*	1.01
Other ethnic group	0.91	0.88	2.40*	0.80
Catholics and Other Christians				
Kembata/Timbaro	0.89	0.79	9.83*	0.23*
Sidama	1.05	1.02	2.48*	0.87
Other ethnic group	1.09	1.11	4.45*	0.86
Protestant Christians				
Hadiya	0.91	0.94	5.59*	0.73
Kembata/Timbaro	0.97	0.88	5.28*	0.51*
Sidama	Ref.	Ref.	Ref.	Ref.
Wolayta	0.94	0.94	3.12*	0.84
Other ethnic group	0.93	0.94	3.88*	0.72
Moslems				
Gurage	1.07	1.10	4.09*	0.21*
Hadiya	0.94	0.76*	2.96*	0.26*
Selite	0.98	1.03	7.86*	0.13*
Other ethnic group	1.05	0.89	3.82*	0.35*
Traditional				
Konta	0.65*	0.70*	3.73*	2.51*
Sidama	0.98	1.08	3.65*	0.74
Other ethnic group	0.67*	0.80	3.35*	1.58*

Continued

	No. Children Ever Born		Ideal Family Size "Up to God"	Family Planning Use/Plan
	Total	In 1991–97		
Marital Homogamy and Group Status				
Same Ethnic, Religion & Language	1.01	1.06	1.06	0.99
Ethnoreligious Majority	1.04	1.07	1.22	1.01
Religious Devotion	1.02	1.01	1.09	1.01
Community Variables				
Ethnoreligious Diversity	1.15*	1.12*	0.29*	1.29*
Urban Residence	0.97	0.83*	1.18	1.06
Family Planning Services	—	—	1.21*	1.35*
Intercept	(1.10)*	(0.66)*	(-0.81)	(-2.05)*
Model Chi-square (df)	1855(33)*	419(35)*	388 (36)*	333 (37)*

Notes: All models control for age at and duration of marriage, spousal age difference, polygynous union and literacy. Logistic model additionally includes number of surviving children, contraceptive knowledge, and spousal family size discussion. Poisson model also controls for number of children ever born before 1991 and experience with child death. * $p \leq 0.05$.

The number of children ever born to a woman varies considerably among the ethnic groups within each religious group (Table 3.6). It also varies by community diversity; the mean number of children ever born increases as community ethnoreligious diversity increases. But the number of children ever born does not systematically vary by marital homogamy or group dominance (Table 3.6). A multivariate poisson model of the number of children ever born, taking into account age and duration of marriage, shows very few ethnoreligious variations in the number of children ever born (Table 3.8). Indeed, the ethnic groups among Moslems and Protestants do not differ. Orthodox Hadiya have fertility that is about 15 percent greater than Hadiya from other religions, and the Konta of all religions tend to be lower. Fertility is unaffected by marital homogamy, community group status, and degree of religiosity (Table 3.8). The positive effect of community ethnoreligious diversity on fertility, however, persists when we introduce control variables in the multivariate model. Recent fertility patterns display the same tendencies (Table 3.8), suggesting that the observed relationships are long-standing in this population.

Compared to other ethnoreligious groups, Moslems of all ethnic groups and the Gurage of all religions are resistant to the idea of contraceptive adoption (Table 3.6). Resistance to contraceptive adoption is especially strong among women who are in a homogamous union, in an ethnoreligious group that is dominant in the community, and in communities with little variation in ethnoreligious identity. The multivariate model (Table 3.8) confirms the very low level of planned contraceptive adoption among the Moslems. The Konta have particularly high levels of planned contraceptive use. Women living in villages or towns with contraceptive services, who have knowledge of more than one method of family planning, and who discuss family size with their husbands have distinctly greater probabilities of contraceptive adoption. Plans to adopt contraceptives are not affected by marital homogamy or by membership to a dominant ethnoreligious group (taking into account husband and wife communication about family size). Community ethnoreligious diversity is, however, strongly associated with an increased likelihood of contraceptive use in the future.

CONCLUSIONS

This chapter has documented the tremendous variability in ethnic and religious group identities in southern Ethiopia. While most observers of this area refer to religious identity and ethnic identity in conflict, this chapter has shown the situation is far more complicated. Using data on the ethnic, religious, and linguistic homogamy of first marriages, we have identified twenty-two distinctive ethnoreligious groups that have a high degree of spousal self-selection, reinforced by geographic concentration. It is not correct to speak of Moslems versus Protestants or other religious comparisons for this population; ethnic groups within each religion vary far too much to make such comparisons valid. Features of marriage and reproduction vary systematically among these ethnoreligious groups. The general tendency is that women in communities in which their ethnoreligious group is dominant, and in which diversity of ethnoreligious identities is low, more often have early marriages with an older husband, and have a husband who has one or more additional wives. These same women also are more likely to believe that their family size is not subject to rational control ("up to God"). In contrast, women living in diverse communities (controlling for urban/rural residence) are more likely to believe that the number of children they have is subject to rational control. Although they display higher fertility patterns, these women are also more likely to plan to use contraceptives. Thus it is community diversity, rather than minority group status, that distinguishes these fertility differences.

These results have several important theoretical implications for understanding ethnic and religious fertility differences in sub-Saharan Africa. The two widely used hypotheses purporting to explain ethnic/religious fertility differentials, the minority-group status and assimilation hypotheses, fail to get empirical support from our study of reproductive behaviors of women in the SNNPR. Taking into account differences in socioeconomic and demographic characteristics and group status, we find enormous ethnoreligious variations in patterns of reproductive preferences, intentions, and behaviors. These persistent differences in reproductive outcomes among ethnoreligious groups may be a component of their *social identity* rather than their response to their minority-group or socioeconomic status. Thus, our results support the cultural hypothesis, which attributes differentials in fertility behavior to cultural factors such as differences in social norms and preferences about appropriate age at marriage, family size, or contraceptive use. Differences in socioeconomic status among ethnoreligious groups may change over time; but these changes may not necessarily eradicate important cultural traditions and psychological traits that define a distinct social identity.

The results of this study also have important policy implications. Perhaps the most important policy-relevant finding is that neither ethnoreligious group dominance, religiosity, nor community diversity is an obstacle for efforts to promote fertility limitation practices in the SNNPR. Moreover, community diversity, rather than being an inhibiting factor, appears to be strongly associated with key ingredients for reproductive preferences, attitudes, and behavior that will lead to lowered fertility.

In keeping with this emphasis on community, our analysis provides strong evidence for the important role family planning services play in determining women's fertility desires and their intent to use contraceptives. In communities where family planning services are available, these services are associated with the ability of women to rationally control their family size as well as with increased use of or intention to use contraceptives. This finding supports the strategy of providing contraceptive services in health clinics and outreach programs, administered by both governmental and nongovernmental organizations. These services have been important in instilling in women a desire to limit their fertility and to learn about and adopt family planning (Hogan et. al. 1999).

Thus, organizers of efforts to reduce fertility in the SNNPR should be less concerned about ethnic or religious group diversity, size, or degree of religiosity and should focus more strongly on expanding and improving family planning service provision. As in almost every nation that has undergone the transition to lower fertility during the late twentieth century, access to family planning is essential. Moreover, as we argued elsewhere (Hogan et al. 1999), government development efforts should also place a high priority on the continuation and strengthening of adult literacy programs offered in recent years and a guarantee of primary schooling for girls. The promotion of economic activities by women also helps to improve both women's status and their family economic situations (Hogan et al. 1999). Combined together these three factors can be a powerful means of engaging the population and moving it toward lowered fertility.

NOTES

The 1997 Community and Family Survey (CFS) of the Southern Nations, Nationalities, and People's Region of Ethiopia was a collaborative project of the Demographic Training and Reseach Center (DTRC) of Addis Ababa University and the Population Studies and Training Center of Brown University, with major funding from the Andrew W. Mellon Foundation. Support for this project was provided by grants from the Compton Foundation, the Packard Foundation, and the Mellon Foundations, and by a Population Council fellowship to Betemariam Berhanu. An earlier version of this chapter was presented at the annual meeting of the Population Association of America, March 23–25, 2000, Los Angeles, California.

1. Although they do not practice any of the Christian or Islam religions, Traditionals (i.e., people who adhere to traditional worship) in the SNNPR fast and pray like those in other religions.

2. In the model that predicts age at first marriage, we control for current age of the respondent to capture the women's cohort experience, an indicator of whether the respondent and her husband were from the same village or town as measures of mobility of the respondents, and place of birth to capture the effects of origin of residence. In modeling spousal age difference we use husband's age instead of the age of the wife because preliminary analysis showed that husband's age explains more variation. We also include husband's literacy status in this model. In addition, we control for literacy status

of the wife, duration of marriage, number of children ever born or surviving, and experience with child death, and the proportion of the majority ethnoreligious group in a community in all the models to control for the size of the group.

The following additional variables were included in our model of contraceptive adoption: husband-wife communication about family planning during the year preceding the survey, desire for additional children as a proxy for motivation for fertility regulation (want to Limit/Space versus Want more), and knowledge of modern contraceptive measures. To overcome the problem of reverse causation between knowledge and ever use of contraceptives, we code the knowledge variable as 0 = knowledge of no methods or of one method, 2 = knowledge of two or three methods, and 3 = knowledge of four methods or more (Hogan et al. 1999; DeGraff 1991).

3. We apply sampling weights to all calculations in the descriptive analysis. The multivariate results are, however, unweighted.

REFERENCES

Agresti, A. (1996). *An Introduction to Categorical Data Analysis.* New York: Wiley.

Bongaarts, J., and S.C. Watkins. (1996). Social interactions and contemporary fertility transitions. *Population and Development Review* 22: 639–682.

BOPED (1996). *A Socio-Economic Profile.* Bureau of Planning and Economic Development, SNNP Regional Government, Awassa, Ethiopia.

Bott, E. (1971). *Family and Social Network; Roles, Norms, and External Relationships in Ordinary Urban Families.* 2nd ed. New York: Free Press.

Boye, A., K. Hill, S. Isaacs, and D. Gordis. (1991). Marriage law and practice in the Sahel. *Studies in Family Planning* 22: 343–349.

Casterline, J.B., L. Williams, and P. McDonald. (1986). The age difference between spouses: Variations among developing countries. *Population Studies* 40: 353–374.

CSA. (1996). *The 1994 Population and Housing Census of Ethiopia; Results for Southern Nations, Nationalities and Peoples' Region. Volume I: Part V. Abridged Statistical Report. Central Statistical Authority.* Addis Ababa, Ethiopia.

DeGraff, D.S. (1991). Increasing contraceptive use in Bangladesh: The role of demand and supply factors. *Demography* 28: 65–81.

DTRC/PSTC. (1998). *Southern Nations, Nationalities, and People's Region—Community and Family Survey: 1997.* Demographic Training and Research Center, Addis Ababa University, and Population Studies and Training Center, Brown University.

Ezeh. A. (1997). Polygyny and reproductive behavior in sub-Saharan Africa: A contextual analysis. *Demography* 34: 355–368.

Forste, R. and M. Tienda. (1996). What's behind racial and ethnic fertility differentials? *Population and Development Review* 22: 109–133. Supplement to *Fertility in the United States: New Patterns, New Theories.*

Goldscheider, C., and W.D. Mosher. (1991). Patterns of contraceptive use in the United States: The importance of religious factors. *Studies in Family Planning* 22: 102–115.

———. (1988). Religious affiliation and contraceptive usage: Changing American patterns, 1955–82. *Studies in Family Planning* 19: 48–57.

Goldscheider, C., and P. Uhlenberg. (1969). Minority group status and fertility. *American Journal of Sciology* 74: 361–372.

Govindasamy, P., and J. DaVanzo. (1992). Ethnicity and fertility differentials in Peninsular Malaysia: Do policies matter? *Population and Development Review* 18: 243–267.

Granovetter, M.S. (1974; 2nd ed. 1995). *Getting a Job: A Study of Contacts and Careers*. Chicago: University of Chicago Press.

Hill, A.G. (ed.). (1985). *Population, Health and Nutrition in the Sahel: Issues in the Welfare of Selected West African Communities*. London, England: KPI.

Hogan, Dennis P., Betemariam Berhanu, and Assefa Hailemariam. (1999). Household organization, women's autonomy, and contraceptive behavior in Southern Ethiopia. *Studies in Family Planning* 30: 303–314.

Jiobu, R., and H. Marshall. (1977). Minority status and family size: A comparison of explanations. *Population Studies* 31: 509–517.

Kollehlon, K.T. (1989). Ethnicity and fertility in Liberia: A test of the minority group status hypothesis. *Social Biology* 36 (1–2): 67–81.

Montgomery, M.R., and J.B. Casterline. (1996). Social learning, social influence, and new models of fertility. *Population and Development Review* 22, Supplement: 151–175.

Mosher, W.D., and C. Goldscheider. (1984). Contraceptive patterns of religious and racial groups in the United States, 1955–76: Convergence and distinctiveness. *Studies in Family Planning* 15: 101–111.

Mosher, W.D., and G.E. Hendershot. (1984). Religion and fertility: A replication. *Demography* 21: 185–191.

Mosher, W.D., D.P. Johnson, and M.C. Horn. (1986). Religion and fertility in the United States: The importance of marriage patterns and Hispanic origin. *Demography* 23: 367–379.

Murty, K.R. and S. De Vos. (1984). Ethnic differences in contraceptive use in Sri Lanka. *Studies in Family Planning* 15(5): 222–232.

Pai Panandiker, V.A., and P. K. Umashankar. (1994). Fertility control and politics in India. *Population and Development Review* 20, Supplement: 89–104.

Pick, J.B., G.L. Tellis, and E.W. Butler. (1989). Fertility determinants in the oil region of Mexico. *Social Biology* 36 (1–2): 45–66.

Ritchey, P.N. (1975). The effect of minority group status on fertility: A re-examination of concepts. *Population Studies* 29: 249–257.

Sly, D.F. (1970). Minority-group status and fertility: An extension of Goldscheider and Uhlenberg. *American Journal of Sociology* 76: 443–459.

Stata Corp. (1999). *Stata Statistical Software: Release 6*. College Station, TX: Stata Corporation.

Stephen, E.H., R.R. Rindfuss, and F.D. Bean. (1988). Racial differences in contraceptive choice: Complexity and implications. *Demography* 25: 53–70.

White, M.J. (1986). Segregation and diversity measures in population distribution. *Population Index* 52: 198–221.

4

THE FERTILITY IMPACT OF THE RAHAD IRRIGATION PROJECT, SUDAN

El-Rayah A. Osman

INTRODUCTION

Research on fertility in developing countries has increased significantly over the past three decades with the initiation of the World Fertility Survey (1970s) and its successor, the Demographic and Health Survey (1980s). Our understanding of fertility has improved considerably as a result of these two extensive surveys. While this research fills an important gap in our knowledge, a conspicuous omission is the lack of studies evaluating the effect of agricultural development projects. The lack of these evaluations means that development planners have missed an opportunity to incorporate features that would enhance desired demographic impacts or reduce those regarded as undesirable.

The main objective of this study is to assess the fertility impact of the Rahad Irrigation Project of central Sudan. Specifically, the study attempts to examine the following questions: (1) Has the Rahad Project influenced women's reproductive behavior through its provision of irrigated land, employment, and social services? (2) Does the presence of the development project at the community level affect the relationship between individual characteristics (e.g., income, occupation) and fertility? (3) Does the Project improve or worsen child survival? The study uses household survey data collected by the author.

Irrigation projects are among the many rural development strategies pursued by the government of Sudan, and many governments in Africa, in order to increase agricultural output and to improve the standards of living of rural people. They do not have specific demographic objectives. However, major irrigation projects may have important demographic impacts, as well as social and economic effects.

The rest of this chapter adopts the following layout. Section two reviews the findings and conceptual and methodological issues of the fertility impact studies conducted in developing countries. Section three describes the project under investigation. The conceptual framework and research hypotheses are discussed in section four. Section five describes the methodology used to collect the data, the research design, and discusses some specification issues. In section six the effect of the Project on fertility is presented. Finally, section seven contains discussion and the conclusions.

AN EVALUATION OF PREVIOUS FERTILITY IMPACT STUDIES

Studies assessing the impact of rural development projects upon fertility in developing countries cover a wide range of projects. They tend to be concentrated in Asia, and cover projects ranging from irrigation, electrification, to integrated rural development projects.[1] The following is a brief review of their findings, methodologies, and policy issues:

First, studies conducted in Asia have established that rural development projects do affect fertility, but results have so far been contradictory. Some studies have found that development projects have pronatalistic effects, and others have found antinatalistic effects, while still others have found no effects. Mueller and Anderson (1982), for example, found that the Comilla Project in Bangladesh had little effect on fertility. The pronatalist influence of the economic aspects of the project (extension services and irrigation) canceled out the antinatalist influence of social factors such as education and family planning. Gosling (1982) found that the Federal Land Development Authority schemes in Malaysia were antinatalist. In Thailand, irrigation exerts a significant negative effect on fertility (Prasith-rathsint et al.1986).

Second, development projects do not influence fertility directly; their impact on fertility is indirect. Specifically, development projects influence the socioeconomic conditions of the population, which affect one or more of the proximate determinants of fertility. Most of the previous fertility impact studies found that rural development projects lead to general improvements in the socioeconomic structure that, in turn, reduce fertility (see, for example, Stoeckel and Jain 1986).

Third, the effects on fertility vary among development projects. Some development projects have more impact on fertility than others. In Thailand, rural electricity projects have a greater impact on fertility than irrigation projects (Prasith-rathsint et al. 1986). In Sri Lanka, combinations of development projects have more impact on fertility than any single project (Sirisena and Stoeckel 1986). Therefore, the more integrated a development intervention is, the greater are its chances of success in influencing fertility.

Fourth, some rural development projects have gender-specific effects on occupation and income. In Sri Lanka, the combined effect of rural electrification, land settlement, and guaranteed price support is to raise male income more than female income (Sirisena and Stoeckel 1986). A policy that is directed at reducing this gender gap in income could contribute to lower fertility. Further, in Malaysia, development projects attract migrants who have lower fertility than nonmigrants (Gosling 1982).

Fifth, whether and to what extent an irrigation project will affect fertility depends on how long it has been in place and how it affects the socioeconomic conditions of the area it serves. Development projects take some time to influence fertility; specification of the time lag after which the effect is discernible is necessary.

Finally, previous fertility impact studies have used cross-sectional designs to evaluate the fertility impact of rural development projects. The classic experimental design is the ideal method, although the quasi-experimental design is usually the only option available to researchers. The ideal design should include observations for both the development project areas and control localities for periods before and after the development project is initiated. Lacking such a design, the researcher could select two parts of the same population, one that has been affected by the development project and one that has not. To further improve the research design, the analyst could use stratification (at the design stage) and statistical controls (at the analysis stage). Stratification and statistical controls reduce the effect of selection bias, which is inherent in evaluating the impact of development projects on fertility. This bias refers to the fact that neither villages nor individuals benefiting from development inputs are selected randomly.

THE RESEARCH SETTING

The Rahad Irrigation Project covers an area about 300 kilometers long and 25 kilometers wide on the east bank of the Rahad River in central Sudan (Fig. 4.1). The Rahad Project is the second largest irrigated agricultural scheme, after Gezira Scheme, in the Sudan. The main purpose of the project is to boost export earnings of medium staple cotton, groundnuts, and sorghum (*dura*). Another goal for the project is to settle and improve the social and economic well-being of the rain-fed cultivators, herders, and nomads inhabiting the area.

In the first phase of the Project, began in 1977, 150,000 *feddans*[2] were irrigated, and by 1981 all areas of the Project had been irrigated. It currently irrigates about 300,000 *feddans* and houses up to 150,000 tenants, residents, and seasonal laborers. The Project area consists of the town of El Fau and forty-six villages, of which ten are preexisting villages incorporated into the Project. Each new village has schools, a health facility, and a filtered potable water system. Depending upon the administrative importance, there may also be corporation offices and staff housing (USAID, 1982).

The Rahad Project recruited its population for resettlement from villages on the Rahad River, from selected villages near the Dinder River, and from areas north of Wad Medani. Each tenant has received a twenty-two *feddans* land tenancy. Eleven *feddans* are for growing cotton and the rest are for the cultivation of groundnuts and sorghum.[3] Sorghum and groundnuts belong to the tenant while the Rahad Corporation markets the cotton. The Project has also allocated 400 tenancies of five *feddans* each in which to grow vegetables and fruits outside the main crop rotation. In addition, the Project allotted 1,296 livestock tenancies of 12 *feddans* each for meat and milk production (Simpson and Simpson 1991).

Fig. 4.1
The Location of the Rahad Irrigation Project

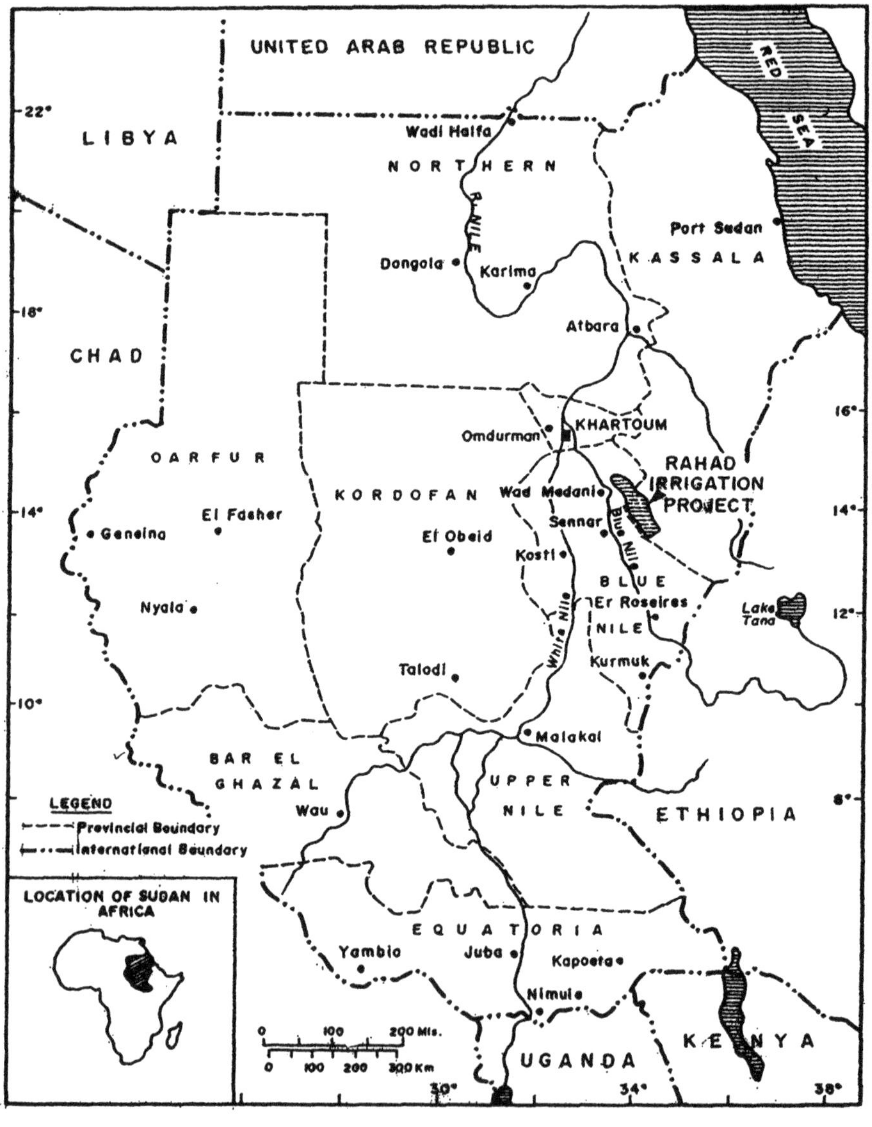

CONCEPTUAL FRAMEWORK AND HYPOTHESES

Conceptual Framework

The conceptual framework of this study (see Fig. 4.2) builds on the general framework developed by Stoeckel and Jain (1986). In this framework, the independent variable (irrigation) influences the dependent variable (fertility) through a number of intervening and intermediate variables. Specifically, rural development projects influence the socioeconomic conditions of the population, and changes in the socioeconomic conditions of the population affect one or more of the proximate determinants of fertility (Davis and Blake 1956; Bongaarts 1978), which influence fertility.

Major irrigation systems can affect fertility by influencing income, labor force participation, and economic productivity. An agricultural irrigation system leads to more effective land use in the following ways: by bringing more land under cultivation, by allowing higher cropping intensity, and by improving farm production, which results in higher household income and wealth. The increases in income and wealth bring more security to agricultural households, allowing them to invest in the health and education of their children. In addition, agricultural irrigation affects labor utilization within the household, opening opportunities for females to participate in the labor force outside the home. The increases in income and female labor force participation are expected to reduce the demand for children. Irrigation brings security and economic prosperity to the community and reduces the risk associated with rain-fed cultivation. In turn, this economic prosperity leads to investment outside the field of agriculture (e.g., rural industries). This investment encourages modernization, which in turn affects desired family size and hence reduces fertility.

Fig. 4.2
Conceptual Framework for the Interrelationship between Irrigation Projects and Fertility

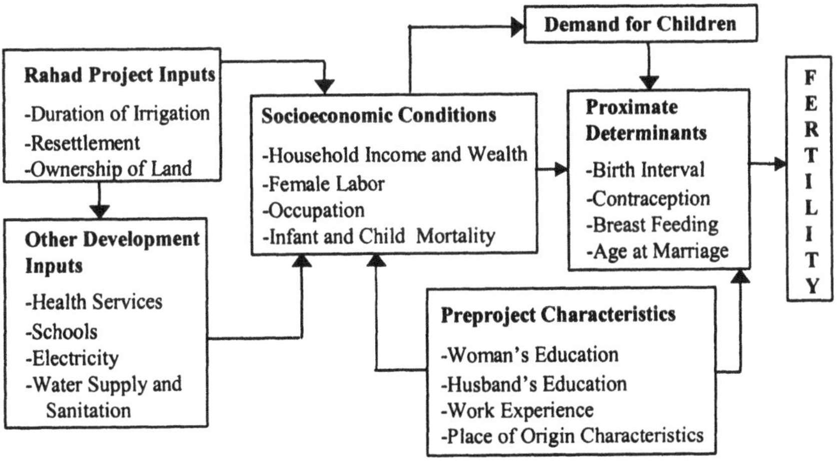

Research Hypotheses

Economic Contributions and Costs of Children

Agricultural development affects fertility by changing the benefits and costs of having children. Rural development projects that include modern agricultural equipment reduce the demand for children's labor by eliminating many of the tasks children customarily perform. Rural development projects also allow parents to invest in the health and education of their children, and this increase in costs motivates parents to curtail their fertility.

The Rahad Project opted for full mechanization of cotton and groundnut production to avoid the classic problems of labor shortage and low production that existed in other irrigated schemes of the Sudan. It also adopted a policy of 100 percent intensive rotation. The labor contribution of children is expected to decline because of mechanization and the higher enrollment of children in schools. I expect the Project to reduce fertility because of the decline in the benefits of large families and the increase in the costs of raising them, other factors being equal.

Income and Fertility

Studies of the determinants of fertility in developing countries have generally found that the effect of income on fertility is ambiguous (Mueller and Short 1983). Holding other factors constant, a rise in income is expected to raise fertility, because parents can afford to have children. Counteracting this is a preference of parents for a higher quality of life for their children. As women's income rises the demand for children tends to decrease, as the time and cost of raising large families become even greater. On the hand, higher incomes also allow for better nutrition and more effective use of social services and medical care, thereby resulting in a rise in fertility, other factors being equal.

The goal of the Project is to increase income and to lessen the risk in income generation. More specifically, its goal is to transform farmers dependent upon animal husbandry and subsistence production of rain-fed sorghum into cash crop farmers dependent on irrigation. The Project has been a success in improving incomes because of mechanization, fertile soil, dynamic structure of management, and adoption of a new accounting system. Thus, in the short run, I expect to find that an increase in household income results in an increase in fertility, other factors being equal.

Availability and Utilization of Social Services and Fertility

Besides individual and household characteristics, fertility is also influenced by the availability of services in the areas in which the women live (Ruiz and Bilsborrow 1988). Availability and utilization of services such as schools, health centers, electricity, and other social services lead to fertility reduction. They allow parents to invest in the quality of life for their children and this entails higher costs. Such services may also impact on fertility by reducing infant and child mortality, thereby reducing the demand for large numbers of children.

One goal of the Project is to improve social well-being through services and facilities that were previously inadequate or nonexistent. I expect to find that the availability and utilization of social services reduce fertility, other factors being constant.

Woman's Roles and Fertility

Three decades ago, Boserup (1970) claimed that agricultural modernization, mechanization, and market integration would lead to a reduction in the economic participation of rural women. She found that in Africa women's participation in the subsistence sector was high, and that agricultural modernization was displacing women. Boserup found that this, in turn, affected their statuses and roles. I argue here that rural development projects provide opportunities for rural women that are not available in nonirrigated areas. Such projects increase their participation in economic activities and eliminate many of the arduous tasks women used to perform. The Rahad Project provides work opportunities for women that are not available in nonirrigated areas and provides work opportunities for women outside the home. I expect the Project to increase female employment outside the home, leading to a reduction in fertility, other factors being equal.

METHODOLOGY

Data and Research Design

The main source of data for the analysis is the fertility and marriage survey conducted by the author in 1993 in the project and the comparison (control) areas. This survey included 1,200 heads of households, 800 from the project and 400 from outside the project, to obtain household data. Within these households, 1,209 ever-married women aged 15–49 years were interviewed, and marriage histories were obtained.[4] A second source of data is village and household data collected in 1975, before the Project began (Galal El Din 1975).

This study uses an ad hoc quasi-experimental design in which two groups were compared after one group was exposed to treatment effects (Cook and Campbell 1979). Since the villages were not randomly assigned to the Project settlements or to the comparison area, the quasi-experimental groups are not necessarily equivalent. However, the villages in the Project and in the comparison area were drawn from the same region. Furthermore, Project and comparison villages were matched on a number of socioeconomic and demographic characteristics to partially rectify the absence of randomization. This study has controlled for preexisting differences among villages using data from Galal El Din's survey (1975) conducted in the pre-Project area. These data also help reduce the selectivity problems inherent in this type of research. The definition and specification of the variables are given in Table 4.1. Descriptive statistics are shown in Table 4.2.

Table 4.1
Description and Specification of the Variables used in the Analysis

Variable	Definition of Variable
PROJECT	A dummy variable having a value of 1 if the woman is living in the project, zero otherwise.
Woman's Characteristics:	
BIRTH5	Live births between 1988 and 1993 adjusted for marriage exposure.
AGE	Age of the woman at the time of the interview (in years).
AGESQ	The square of age.
AGEM	Age of the woman at first marriage (in years).
DEAD10	Number of children died between 1983 and 1993.
DEAD5-15	Number of children died between 1978 and 1988.
EDUC2	A dummy variable having a value of 1 if the woman had completed primary education (1–6 years), 0 otherwise.
EDUC3	A dummy variable having a value of 1 if the woman had completed secondary education and above (7 years or more), 0 otherwise.
CURRENT	A dummy variable having a value of 1 if the woman is currently married, 0 otherwise.
ARAB	A dummy variable having a value of 1 if the woman is from an Arab household, 0 otherwise.
SEPARATION	Duration of spousal separation (months) in the last five years.
HOURS	Number of hours worked last week in all occupations combined.
CHILD5	The number of living children under age 5.
BIRTH10	The number of live births between 1983 and 1993.
Husband's Characteristics:	
HEDUC2	A dummy variable having a value of 1 if the husband had completed primary education, 0 otherwise.
HEDUC3	A dummy variable having a value of 1 if the husband had completed secondary education and above, 0 otherwise.
AGRI	A dummy variable having a value of 1 if the husband's occupation is in agriculture, 0 otherwise.
COMMERCE	A dummy variable having a value of 1 if the husband's occupation is in commerce, 0 otherwise.
Household Characteristics:	
HHAGE	Age of head of the household (years).
HHEDUC2	A dummy variable having a value of 1 if the education of head of the household is primary (1–6 years), 0 otherwise.
HHEDUC3	A dummy variable having a value of 1 if the education of the head of the household is secondary and above (7 years or more), 0 otherwise.
HMEDUC	Average education of household members is the ratio of the number of years of schooling of household members divided by the number of household members aged 7 years and older.

Continued

Variable	Definition of Variable
HMLABOR	Household labor is the ratio of the number of household members who worked last year (aged 10 and over), divided by the number of household members aged 15–65 years.
LAND	Size of landholding by the household (in *feddans*).
EXP	Total annual household expenditure (in Sudanese pounds).
ASSET	Total number of household assets.
RED	A dummy variable having a value of 1 if the construction of the house is red brick, zero otherwise.
SMALL	A dummy variable having a value 1 if the amount of land owned before project is 1–19 *feddans*, zero otherwise.
BIG	A dummy variable having a value of 1 if the amount of land owned before project is 20–650 *feddans*, zero otherwise.
Village Characteristics:	
HEALTH	A dummy variable having a value of 1 if the type of health facility is a hospital or health center, zero otherwise.
WATER	A dummy variable having a value of 1 if the main source of water in the village is piped, zero otherwise.
ELECTRI	A dummy variable having a value of 1 if there is electriity in village, zero otherwise.
Preproject Village Characteristics:	
CWR	The child-woman ratio of the village from which the woman joined the project.
FORMAL	The percent of formal education in preproject village.
POLYGYNY	The percent of polygyny among married male household heads in the preproject village.
SCHOOL	A dummy variable having a value of 1 if there was a school in the preproject village, 0 otherwise.
HSIZE	The average size of the household in the preproject village.

Table 4.2
Descriptive Statistics of Variables Used in the Analysis

Variable	Mean	Standard Deviation	Minimum	Maximum
PROJECT	0.71	0.45	00.00	1.00
Woman's Characteristics:				
BIRTH5	1.68	1.22	00.00	5.00
AGE	31.64	8.50	14.00	49.00
AGESQ	1073.40	561.84	196.00	2401.00
AGEM	16.33	3.45	10.00	37.00
DEAD10	0.30	0.63	00.00	4.00

Continued

Variable	Mean	Standard Deviation	Minimum	Maximum
DEAD5-15	0.27	0.57	00.00	4.00
EDUC2	0.31	0.46	00.00	1.00
EDUC3	0.06	0.23	00.00	1.00
CURRENT	0.94	0.24	00.00	1.00
HOURS	6.64	14.39	00.00	64.00
SEPARATION	0.88	4.37	00.00	60.00
ARAB	0.91	0.29	00.00	1.00
CHILD5	1.15	0.89	00.00	3.00
BIRTH10	2.85	1.73	00.00	8.00
Husband's Characteristics:				
HEDUC2	0.42	0.49	00.00	1.00
HEDUC3	0.15	0.35	00.00	1.00
AGRI	0.59	0.49	00.00	1.00
COMMERCE	0.16	0.36	00.00	1.00
Household Characteristics:				
HHAGE	44 .03	11.77	18.00	73.00
HHEDUC2	0.40	0.49	00.00	1.00
HHEDUC3	0.40	0.35	00.00	1.00
HMEDUC	3.23	2.07	00.00	17.50
HMLABOR	0.56	0.43	00.11	2.00
SMALL	0.30	0.46	00.00	1.00
BIG	0.27	0.44	00.00	1.00
RED	0.44	0.50	00.00	1.00
LAND	14.12	18.12	00.00	430.00
EXP	12.23	0.53	10.00	15.47
ASSET	0.95	1.13	00.00	10.00
Village Characteristics:				
WATER	0.71	0.45	00.00	1.00
HEALTH	0.27	0.44	00.00	1.00
ELECTRIC	0.18	0.39	00.00	1.00
Preproject Village Characteristics:				
CWR	7.34	5.37	01.25	44.59
FORMAL	27.24	27.26	02.00	70.00
POLYGYNY	4.63	3.09	02.00	25.00
HSIZE	4.19	2.08	03.80	13.70
SCHOOL	0.43	0.50	00.00	1.00

Specification Issues

This section examines the fertility impact of the Project on fertility using a simultaneous-equation system (multiequation) involving infant and child mortality, household income, and female labor force participation as endogenous variables. The simultaneity is exhibited in the various decisions taken by households in developing countries (Keeley 1975). Moreover, because we are interested in the direct effect of the project on income, mortality, and female labor force participation, this framework allows us to examine the association among several key household decisions. Analysis of these interdependent household decisions may help to clarify efficient policies for rural development. In addition to allowing for interdependency and simultaneity, we also need to adjust for selection bias, because neither the villages nor the individuals were selected randomly into the project.

Fertility Equation:

$$BIRTH5= a_0 + a_1 AGE + a_2 AGESQ + a_3 AGEM + a_4 DEAD5\text{-}15 + a_5 EDUC2 + a_6 EDUC3 + a_7 HOURS + a_8 HEDUC2 + a_9 HEDUC3 + a_{10} AGRI + a_{11} COMMERCE + a_{12} SEPARATION + a_{13} EXP + a_{14} PROJECT + \mu_1 \quad (1)$$

where μ_1 is an error term.

The dependent variable in equation (1) is the number of live births in the five years before the survey was conducted, that is, 1988 to 1993.[5] A measure of recent fertility is used to allow enough time for the project to influence fertility.[6] This measure is also intended to minimize recall error.

A number of variables are introduced as control variables in equation (1): age and age squared are included to control for fecundity; age at first marriage, which reflects exposure of the woman to intercourse; child survival, which has biological and behavioral effects (Preston 1976); schooling, known to have pervasive effects on fertility (Bledose et al. 1999); female employment,[7] which increases the costs of raising children; husband's education and occupation; total annual household expenditure, a proxy for household income (Ainsworth 1989); and spousal separation, which can reduce fertility (Millman and Potter 1984). The main variable of interest in equation (1) is participation (or nonparticipation) in the project, and is used to evaluate the impact of the project on fertility.

We note that in this study fertility differentials are examined in a specific period (1988–1993). No claim can be made about the size and direction of the project effects on fertility outside this reference period. We assume here that the project effects on fertility occur with certain lags. Specifically, we focus on fertility differentials after the project has been in place for ten to fifteen years.

Mortality (child deaths) Equation:

$$DEAD10 = b_0 + b_1 AGE + b_2 EDUC2 + b_3 EDUC3 + b_4 HEDUC2 + b_5 HEDUC3 + b_6 BIRTH10 + b_7 EXP + b_8 RED + b_9 WATER + b_{10} ELECTRI + b_{11} HEALTH + b_{12} PROJECT + \mu_2 \quad (2)$$

where μ_2 is an error term.

The dependent variable in the mortality equation is the number of dead children in the ten years preceding the survey (1983–1993). It is used as a proxy for the probability of child mortality, which is the most commonly used dependent variable in mortality analysis.

Child survival is affected by a number of factors: maternal age, which affects the mother's health and ability to provide adequate nutrition to the fetus and to the infant; the level of education of both parents is of critical importance to child survival (Farah and Preston 1982); the number of live births born to the woman, which measures the effect of reproductive behavior; total annual household expenditure, a proxy for household income, which increases the use of health care and other services (Casterline et al. 1989); socioeconomic status of the household, measured by the amount of land owned by the household, and the types of dwellings; and the availability of social services, which influences the health and survival of children.[8] The effect of the Project on child mortality is also of interest. The canal system built in these projects leads to waterborne diseases such as schistosomiasis, malaria, and diarrheal diseases (Bradley 1985).

Female Employment Equation:

HOURS= c_0+ c_1 AGE +c_2 EDUC2 + c_3 EDUC3 + c_4 HEDUC2 + c_5 HEDUC3 + c_6 ARAB + c_7 CURRENT + c_8 EXP + c_9 LAND + c_{10} CHILD5 + c_{11} PROJECT + μ_3

where μ_3 is an error term (3)

The dependent variable in the female employment equation is the number of hours worked last week; it is usually taken as a measure of current employment.[9]

A number of variables are introduced as control variables in the female employment equation: age, which reflects changes in the opportunity structure and cohort effects; level of education, which influences the skill levels women bring to the labor market; marital status, where the presence of a husband means the availability of a source of income that reduces the need for the woman to work; husband's education; maternal status; ethnicity, a proxy for cultural factors (see Anker and Knowles 1979); ownership of land or the availability of land, which induces women to join the labor force; and annual household expenditure, a proxy for household income, which measures the economic status of the household. Rural development projects provide work opportunities for women that are not available elsewhere. They increase their participation in the labor force, and eliminate many difficult tasks women used to perform. The Rahad Project expanded work opportunities and offered a wage market for women that is not available in nonirrigated areas.

Income Equation:

EXP= d_0+ d_1 HHAGE + d_2 HHEDUC2 + d_3 HHEDUC3 + d_4 HMEDUC + d_5 HMLABOR + d_6 LAND + d_7 ASSET + d8 ROJECT +μ_4

where μ_4 is an error term (4)

The dependent variable in the income equation is the total annual household expenditure, a proxy for household income. Household income is affected by a number of factors: age and the educational level of the head of the household; the labor force participation of household members; the amount of land owned by the members of the household, which is an important source of income; and household assets. An agricultural irrigation system leads to effective land use by bringing more land under cultivation. It allows higher cropping intensity and improves farm production, resulting in higher household income.

Selection Equation:

$$PROJECT = e_0 + e_1\ EDUC2 + e_2\ EDUC3 + e_3\ HEDUC2 + e_4\ HEDUC3 + e_5\ SMALL + e_6\ BIG + e_7\ CWR + e_8\ FORMAL + e_9\ PLOYGMY + e_{10}\ HSIZE + e_{11}\ SCHOOL + \mu_5$$

where μ_5 is an error term (5)

Adjustment for selection bias is critical since neither the villages nor individuals are randomly selected for the Project (Heckman 1979). The selection of a village for inclusion in the Project was based on a number of factors, including technical consideration (such as the possibility for irrigation) and the availability of land. Ownership of land before the project and experience in agriculture led to the selection of certain people but not others. Therefore, modeling of the selection process is vital to achieve valid estimates of the project's effect on fertility.

The dependent variable in the selection equation is the woman's current place of residence: project or nonproject (control). A number of variables are included in the selection equation to control for the preproject characteristics of the respondents. Two individual-level variables—the educational levels of the wife and her husband—are important factors in the selection process, not only in the initial decision to join the project, but also in the extent to which couples benefit from the project. Participation in the development project requires resettlement into new locations, interactions with new ethnic groups, and a change in lifestyle. Education gives the individual more options; it facilitates the acquisition of information and allows the individual to take risks based on available knowledge. The amount of land owned by the household before the project began and the average household size in the preproject village are also included in the selection equation.[10] Finally, four village-level variables are included in the selection equation: the child-woman Ratio, the percent of polygamy among male heads of households, the presence of a school, and the percent of educated persons in the preproject location. The use of these village-level variables would allow us to control for preproject differences between project and nonproject.

ESTIMATION ISSUES AND EMPIRICAL EVIDENCE

Estimation Issues and Results

The model employed to estimate the effect of the project on fertility as described in the above equations has an interactive feature; that is, key household decisions are simultaneously made. Moreover, we modeled the assignment process to achieve valid estimates of the effects of the project on fertility. This type of framework precludes the use of ordinary least squares (see Maddala 1983; Greene 1997). Among the available methods of estimation, we prefer two-stage least squares (2SLS) because it yields consistent and unbiased estimates of the parameters. It is obtained by entering the predicted values of the endogenous variables as independent variables in the second stage (Johnston 1984).

The unit of analysis in this study is the individual woman. The sample consists of 1,134 ever-married women who were interviewed in eleven villages irrigated by the Rahad Project and in six nonirrigated villages. The results of the 2SLS estimation are presented in Table 4.3, with the correction for selection bias. Table 4.4 reports the indirect effects of the project on the dependent variables.[11]

Empirical Evidence: The Effect of the Project on Fertility

Figure 4.3 compares recent fertility between the project (where inputs of irrigation, intensification, and mechanization are dominant) and the control area (where rain-fed cultivation, animal husbandry and labor migration are dominant). The level of fertility was high in both the project and the comparison area, but somewhat higher in the project area. The higher fertility in the project may be attributed, in part, to the need for children to help in farming activities, to the relative availability of health services, and to the increase in income due to the project.

Table 4.3
2SLS Regression Results for Fertility, Mortality, Employment, and Income with Correction for Selection Bias

Explanatory Variable	Selection Equation	BIRTH5 (1)	DEAD10 (2)	HOURS (3)	EXP (4)
Project: No		—	—	—	—
Yes		0.498*	-0.244*	5.859*	0.012
Woman's Characteristics:					
Age		0.207*	0.001	0.460*	
Age Squared		-0.004*			
Age at First Marriage		-0.023**			
Mortality (DEAD5-15)		0.327*			
Fertility (BIRTH10)			0.127*		

Continued

Explanatory Variable	Selection Equation	BIRTH5 (1)	DEAD10 (2)	HOURS (3)	EXP (4)
Wife's Education:					
No education	—	—	—	—	
Primary	-0.103	-0.027	-0.080***	-0.598	
Secondary and above	-0.390***	0.049	-0.125**	6.636*	
Hours Worked Last Week		-0.011*			
Marital Status:					
Divorced or Widowed				—	
Currently Married				-7.450*	
Ethnicity: Non-Arab				—	
Arab				-6.307*	
Living Children under Age 5				-0.560	
Spousal Separation (months)		-0.019*			
Husband's Characteristics:					
Husband's Education:					
No education	—	—	—	—	
Primary	-0.024	0.017	-0.030	0.037	
Secondary and above	-0.328**	-0.051	-0.015	-0.544	
Husband's Occupation: Other		—			
Agriculture		0.066			
Commerce		0.108			
Household Characteristics:					
Age of Head of Household					0.002***
Education of Head:					
No Education					—
Primary					-0.005
Secondary and above					0.006
Education of Household Members (HMEDUC)					0.036*
Household Labor (HMLABOR)					0.334*
Annual Household Expenditure (Ln Ls)		0.274**	-0.117***	-8.967*	
Landholding Size by the Household (*feddans*)				0.094*	0.009*
Household Assets					0.138*
Type of Dwelling: Other			—		
Fire Bricks (RED)			-0.037		
Village Characteristics:					
Main Source of Water Supply In Village: Other			—		
Piped			-0.039		
Electricity in Village: No			—		
Yes			-0.121**		
Type of Health Facility in Village: DS+S			—		
H+HC			-0.028		
Preproject Village Characteristics:					
CWR in Preproject Village	-0.016				
% of Polygyny in Preproject Village	0.114*				

Continued

Explanatory Variable	Selection Equation	BIRTH5 (1)	DEAD10 (2)	HOURS (3)	EXP (4)
% Formal Education in Preproject Village	-0.007**				
Average Household Size in Preproject Village	-0.333*				
School in Preproject Village: No	—				
Yes	0.632*				
Size of Landholding before Project: Landless	—				
Small (1–19 *feddans*)	-1.034*				
Big (more than 20 *feddans*)	-0.297*				
Lambda		-0.199**	0.042	-1.728	0.067
Constant	2.158	-4.538	1.610	109.49	11.965
N	1134	1134	1134	1134	1134

* $p < 0.01$ ** $p < 0.05$ *** $p < 0.10$. — Reference or omitted category.

Table 4.4
Indirect and Total Effects of the Project on Fertility

	Direct	Indirect	Total
Fertility	0.498	-0.141	0.357
Mortality	-0.244	0.062	-0.182
Employment	5.859	-0.387	5.472
Income	0.012	—	0.012

Source: Calculated from Table 4.3.

Table 4.3 shows that participation in the development project increased fertility within the last five years. Specifically, in the five years before the survey, women in the project had 0.498 live births more than women in nonirrigated areas. One reason for this unexpected result is the low level of contraceptive use in the sample. It is not the policy of the project to encourage the use of contraception. More fundamentally, this finding of a pronatal effect of the project may reflect the relative availability of health services and the low cost of raising children (free schooling and low fees in the project area) as well as the high benefits of having children (through child labor). Mechanization and the increased size of land raise income, and this too may increase fertility. Temporary spousal separation is another important factor. The frequency of spousal separation was lower in the project than in the control area. There is also evidence of higher marital instability among women in the control area compared to those in the project.

Fig. 4.3
Number of Live Births in the Five Years Before the Survey, by Project and Control Areas (Ever-Married Women Age 15-49)

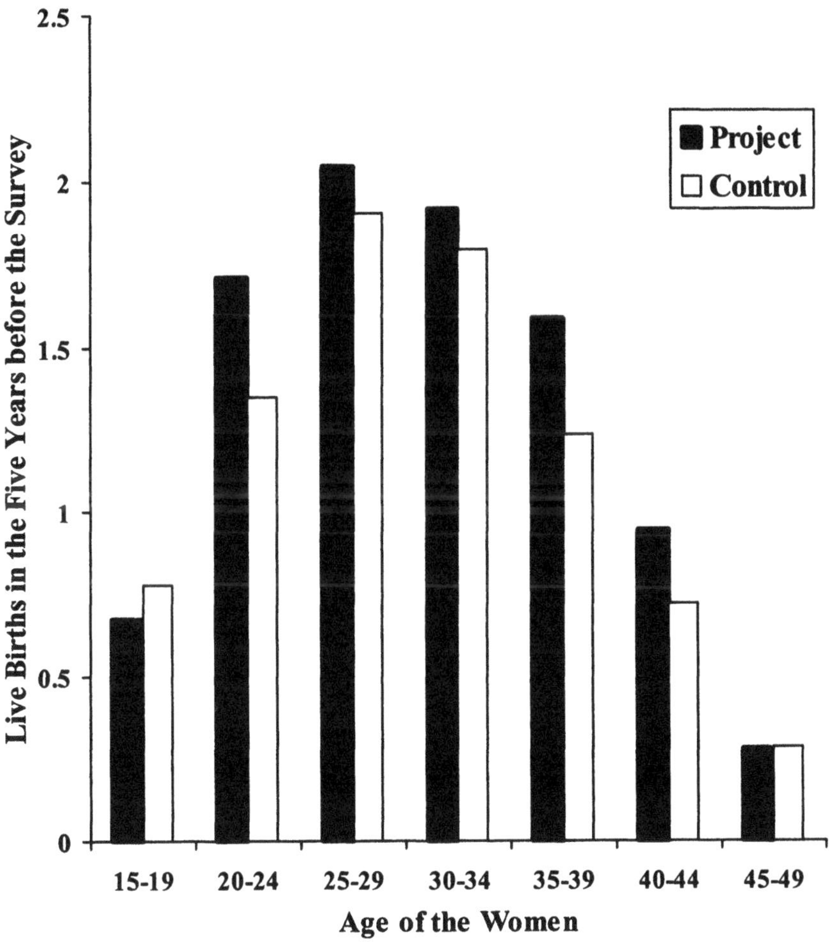

These findings are consistent with other research that also found that at early stage of modernization, fertility may increase (Nag 1980). However, taking into account the indirect effect of the project on fertility (through child mortality, female employment, and household income), the project's effect on fertility is reduced to 0.357 live births (see Table 4.4). This means that by ignoring the indirect effects we are overestimating the effect of the project on fertility.

Note that the variable lambda, an indicator of the presence or nonpresence of selection bias, has a negative coefficient and is statistically significant (bottom of Table 4.3). This means that, controlling for other variables, the project attracted women with lower fertility. The fact that lambda is statistically significant indicates that selection bias is present and has an effect on fertility. (A comparison of results with and without the adjustment for selection bias reveals that ignoring the selection bias leads to an underestimation of the effect of the project on fertility.)

Participation in the development project also has a significant effect on child mortality. In the ten years before the survey, women in the Rahad Project had 0.244 fewer child deaths compared to women in the control area. This finding may be attributed, in part, to the availability of health services in the project area compared to the comparison area. The results indicate that the indirect effect of the project on child mortality, operating through fertility and household income, is 0.062.

Participation in the Rahad Project increases female employment. In the week before the survey was conducted, women in the development project worked 5.8 hours more than women in the control area. Thus, the Rahad Project expanded work opportunities. However, when considering the indirect effect of the project on female employment (operating through fertility and household income), the effect of the project on female employment is reduced slightly.

Finally, participation in the development project raises household income, but the effect is not statistically significant. No indirect effects of the development project on household income are built into the model.

The above findings point to the important effects of development interventions on socioeconomic and demographic variables. The results support the contention that development projects affect fertility by changing the socioeconomic structure. Specifically, participation in the development project increases recent fertility, reduces child mortality, expands employment opportunities for women, and improves the general standard of living. Consideration of the indirect effects of the project on fertility (those operating through child mortality, female employment, and household income) reduces the estimated effect of the project on fertility, as well as on the other dependent variables. Finally, ignoring the selection bias in fertility impact studies would cause us to substantially underestimate the effect of the project on fertility, as well as on the other endogenous variables. This finding raises serious doubts about the validity of the results of many previous fertility impact studies.

DISCUSSION AND CONCLUSION

In this study, we assess the fertility effect of the Rahad Irrigation Project of central Sudan, using microeconomic data collected by the investigator from rural Rahad. The assessment employs a simultaneous-equation system involving mortality, income, and employment as the other endogenous variables. This modeling approach allows us to examine the interactions of several key household decisions. The estimation method is two-stage least sqaures (2SLS). The estimation also includes an adjustment for selection bias (i.e., selection into the project).

The key results are as follows. First, participation in the development project increases recent fertility. This finding may be attributed to the low level of contraceptive use in the study area, to the relative availability of health services, to the low cost of raising children, and or to the lack of opportunities open to women. These all reflect the low status of women in this setting. This finding has important policy implication. The rise in fertility may nullify the economic improvement achieved by participating in the development project, thus jeopardizing the goals of the project. Consideration of this fertility increase helps promote consistency between the goals of population policy and development policy.

We need to repeat here that we have examined the effects of the projects on fertility in a specific period (1988–1993). We assume that the effects of the project on fertility occur with certain lags. This means we did not examine the cumulative effect of the project on fertility since it has been in place, rather we focused on differentials in a certain period. Therefore, we cannot claim anything about the direction and size of the project effects on fertility outside the five-year reference period.

Second, participation in the development project significantly reduces child deaths. This may be due in part to the relative availability of social services, and in particular to health services in the project area. This finding has major policy implications. Apart from the need to reduce human suffering, a reduction in child mortality is widely believed to be a prerequisite for lower fertility. We must note, however, that the establishment of irrigation projects may lead to waterborne diseases such as malaria, bilharzia, and diarrheal diseases. A considerable effort is needed to combat these public health problems using cost-effective strategies.

Third, participation in the development project offers employment opportunities for rural women that are not available elsewhere. This finding is inconsistent with the research of Boserup (1970), who claimed that agricultural modernization, mechanization, and market integration would reduce participation of women in the labor force.

Fourth, taking into account the indirect effects of the development projects on fertility (through mortality, employment, and income) reduces the magnitude of the estimated effect. Consideration of the indirect and interdependent household decisions helps clarify efficient policies for rural development.

Finally, the results also revealed that significant selection processes are at work. Had we ignored the selection bias in this nonrandomized study, the effect of the development project on fertility would have been substantially underestimated. This finding raises questions about the validity of the many previous fertility studies that did not account explicitly for selection bias. Adjusting for selection bias is crucial in any quasi-experimental design since subjects are not assigned randomly.

Our estimates show that the project increased fertility in the period under consideration, and also that substantial selection processes are at work. The implication is that in settings where children are highly valued and fertility desires are high—a setting common in Africa—agricultural irrigation projects that provide access to land, employment, income, and health services can have a pronatalist effect. Counteracting this requires accompanying development projects with family planning programs and other antinatalist efforts. Otherwise, the short-term effects of social services provided by rural development projects would be to increase the rate of population growth.

NOTES

This chapter is based on my doctoral work at Brown University. I wish to express my sincere appreciation to John Casterline, who provided advice, suggestions, ideas, and support. I would also like to thank Michael White, Roger Avery, Samuel Agyei-Mensah, and Carol Apt for their helpful comments. The Population Studies and Training Center at Brown University supported the fieldwork with funds provided by the Mellon Foundation. I gratefully acknowledge assistance from the United Nations Fund for Population Activities (UNFPA) and the Rockefeller Foundation.

1. See Barlow (1982); Bilsborrow and Delargy (1985); Jain (1982); Oberai (1992); Robinson and Kantner (1988); Ruiz and Bilsborrow (1988); Stoeckel and Jain (1986); United Nations (1988); and Vlassoff and Khuda (1988).
2. One *feddan* is equal to 1.04 acres.
3. The tenancy is a nontransferable, nonmortgagable farming unit registered in the name of the head of the household. Families who have held traditional land rights of more than 22 *feddans* received a number of tenancies on condition that each tenancy had to be registered under a different name. Landowners in the Project area received the highest priority in the awarding of land tenancies, followed by residents of the area who practiced agricultural activities, followed by all other residents. Other qualified Sudanese involved or noninvolved in the project received the lowest priority in the allotment of tenancies (USAID 1982).
4. The sample design was as follows. In the Project, the villages were stratified on the following factors: the date of establishment of the village, its administrative importance, whether the village is incorporated or newly established by the Project, and the availability of health and education services. Eleven villages were then randomly selected from the Project—eight new villages and three preexisting villages incorporated by the Project. In the control area, the villages were stratified into three categories: high, medium, and low, on the basis of availability of health and education services. Six villages were randomly selected from the nonirrigated villages.
5. I constructed an "exposure" variable whereby women who are recently married (in the year before the survey) and women who are widowed or divorced in the five years preceding the survey were excluded. Seventy-five cases were omitted and 1,134 observations were used in the analysis. The number of live births in the five years before the survey was conducted is divided by the exposure variable and multiplied by five. The exposure variable ranges from one to five.
6. A measure of recent fertility is preferred over a lifetime measure because participation in the Project varies between sixteen years (for those women who joined the Project in 1977) and twelve years (for those who joined the Project in 1981).
7. Female employment is defined as the number of hours worked the week before the survey was conducted in all occupation combined, and is measured as a continuous

variable. It is assumed that if a woman worked in the previous week, she is more likely to have worked in the previous year. The correlation between working last year and number of hours worked last week is high (0.78).

8. Social services include schools, electricity, and health care facilities. We need to note that the presence of electricity in a village does not assume that all households have electricity, or that those who do were connected on the same date. Similarly, we also need to note that the presence of a school or health facility does not indicate anything about the quality of the services provided or when the facility or service was established.

9. See note no. 7 above.

10. The size of land owned by the household was selected because it affects the individual's likelihood of joining or being selected into the project, yet it has no direct relationship to recent fertility (Moffitt 1991).

11. These indirect effects are rough approximations computed by using the estimation method below. The precise calculation of indirect effects would require the use of matching dependent and independent variables. This is not possible, however, since births in the last five years cannot logically be used to predict deaths in the last ten years. The indirect effects (see Cohen and Cohen 1983) of the project on fertility with correction for selection bias (see Table 4.4) are estimated as follows:

Indirect effect: (-0.244) (0.327) + (5.859) (-0.011) + (0.012) (0.0274) = -0.141.
Total effect: direct effect + indirect effect = 0.498 - 0.144 = 0.357.

REFERENCES

Ainsworth, M. (1989). Socioeconomic determinants of fertility in Ivory Coast. Living Standards Measurement Study. Working Paper 53. World Bank.

Anker, R., and J. Knowles. (1979). A micro-analysis of female labor force participation. Pp. 137–176 in G. Standing and G. Sheehan (eds.). *Labor Force Participation in Low Income Countries.* Geneva: ILO.

Barlow, R. (ed.). (1982). *Case Studies in the Demographic Impact of Asian Development Projects.* Ann Arbor: Center for Research on Economic Development, University of Michigan.

Bilsborrow, R., and P. Delargy. (eds.). (1985). *Impact of Rural Development on Demographic Behavior.* Population Development Studies, No. 9. New York: UNFPA.

Bledose, C., et al. (eds.). (1999). *Critical Perspectives on Schooling and Fertility in the Developing World.* Washington, DC.: National Academy Press.

Bongaarts, J. (1978). A framework for analyzing the proximate determinants of fertility. *Population and Development Review* 4: 105–132.

Boserup, E. (1970). *Woman's Role in Economic Development.* New York: St. Martin's.

Bradley, D. (ed.). (1985). The blue nile health project: A comprehensive approach to the prevention and control of water-associated diseases in irrigated schemes of the Sudan. *Journal of Tropical Medicine and Hygiene* (special issue) No. 88.

Casterline, J., et al. (1989). Household income and child survival in Egypt. *Demography* 26: 15–35.

Cohen, J., and P. Cohen. (1983). *Applied Multiple Regression/Correlation Analysis for the Behavioral Sciences.* Hillsdale, NJ: Lawrence Erlbaum.

Cook, T., and D. Campbell. (1979). *Quasi-experimentation: Design and Analysis Issues for Field Settings.* Boston: Houghton Mifflin Company.

Davis, K., and J. Blake. (1956). Social structure and fertility: An analytical framework. *Economic Development and Cultural Change* 4: 211–235.

Farah, A., and S. Preston. (1982). Child mortality in the Sudan. *Population and Development Review* 2: 365–383.

Galal El Din, M. (1975). *The Human Factor in the Rahad Project Area: Phase I Results of Population and Socioeconomic Survey.* Khartoum: Government Printing Press.

Gosling, P. (1982). The demographic implications of agricultural land settlements: A case study of Malaysia FELDA (Federal Land Development) schemes. Pp. 59–100 in R. Barlow (ed.). *Case Studies in the Demographic Impact of Asian Development Projects.*

Greene, W. (1997). *Econometric Analysis.* 3rd ed. Upper Saddle River, NJ: Prentice-Hall.

Heckman, J. (1979). Sample selection bias as a specification error. *Econmetrica* 47: 153–161.

Jain, A. (1982). *Fertility Implications of USAID Development Assistance to India.* New York: The Population Council.

Johnston, J. (1984). *Econometrics Methods.* 2nd ed. New York: McGraw-Hill.

Keeley, M. (1975). A comment on an interpretation of the economic theory of fertility. *Journal of Economic Literature* 13: 461–468.

Maddala, G. (1983). *Limited-dependent Variables and Qualitative Variables in Econometrics.* Cambridge: Cambridge University Press.

Millman, S., and R. Potter. (1984). The fertility impact of spousal separation. *Studies in Family Planning* 15: 121–126.

Moffitt, R. (1991). Program evaluation with non-experimental data. *Evaluation Review* 15: 291–314.

Mueller, E., and J. Anderson. (1982). The economic and demographic impact of the Comilla project in Bangladesh: A case study. Pp. 1–57 in R. Barlow (ed.). *Case Studies in the Demographic Impact of Asian Development Projects.*

Mueller, E., and K. Short. (1983). Effect of income and wealth on the demand for children. Pp. 590–635 in R. Bulatao and R. Lee (eds.). *Determinants of Fertility in Developing Countries.* New York: Academic Press.

Nag, M. (1980). How modernization can also increase fertility. *Current Anthropology* 21: 571–587.

Oberai, A. (1992). *Assessing the Demographic Impact of Development Projects: Conceptual, Methodological and Policy Issues.* Geneva: ILO.

Prasith-rathsint, S. et al. (1986). Fertility effects of agricultural irrigation in northeastern Thailand. Pp. 73–84 in J. Stoeckel and A. Jain (eds.). *Fertility in Asia: Assessing the Impact of Development Projects.*

Preston, S. (1976). Introduction. Pp. 1–18 in S. Preston (ed.). *The Effects of Infant and Child Mortality on Fertility.* New York. Academic Press.

Robinson, W., and J. Kantner. (1988). The impact of development programs on fertility: A framework for analysis. *Asia-Pacific Population Journal* 3: 65–80.

Ruiz, L., and R. Bilsborrow. (1988). Demographic effect of rural development projects: A case study of Ecuador. Carolina Population Center Papers No. 26.

Simpson, I., and M. Simpson. (1991). Systems of agricultural production in central Sudan and Khartoum. Pp. 242–279 in G. Craig (ed.). *The Agriculture of the Sudan.* Oxford: Oxford University Press.

Sirisena, N., and J. Stoeckel. (1986). Fertility impacts of development programs in Sri Lanka. Pp. 25–54 in J. Stoeckel and A. Jain (eds.). *Fertility in Asia: Assessing the Impact of Development Projects.*

Stoeckel, J., and A. Jain. (eds.). (1986). *Fertility in Asia: Assessing the Impact of Development Projects.* London: Fruter Press.

United Nations. (1988). *Assessing the Demographic Consequences of Major Development Projects.* Proceedings of a United Nations Workshop. New York, December 1–4, 1986. Study No. 81.

USAID. (1982). *Sudan: The Rahad Irrigation Project.* Project Impact Evaluation Report No. 31.

Vlassoff, C., and B. Khuda. (eds.). (1988). *Impact of Modernization on Development and Demographic Behavior: Case Studies in Seven Developing Countries.* Ottawa: IDRC.

5

SOCIAL SETTING, BIRTH TIMING, AND SUBSEQUENT FERTILITY IN THE GHANAIAN SOUTH

Samuel Agyei-Mensah, Asbjorn Aase and Kofi Awusabo-Asare

INTRODUCTION

It has long been recognized that the timing of first births has implications for lifetime fertility. Studies conducted in the United States during the 1970s and 1980s found evidence linking early childbearing to subsequent high completed fertility (see, for instance, Trussell and Menken 1978). Other evidence, however, suggests that early childbearing does not necessarily lead to subsequent high fertility (see Davis and Blake 1956). Morgan and Rindfuss (1999) found in an analysis of recent U.S. data that women who begin childbearing early have more children during their lifetimes, but this differential is now substantially less than it was for earlier birth cohorts. Similarly, it has been observed that early child-bearing still remains common in much of the developing world, though fertility is falling (Althaus 1991).

This chapter deals with the link between the timing of first birth and subsequent fertility in Ghana and examines the factors—especially the contextual factors—that condition this relationship. Our analytical strategy is to compare three birth cohorts of women—born in the 1950s, 1960s, and 1970s, respectively—resident in five distinct communities drawn from three settlements in the country. In many respects, the data represent a marked departure from data used in prior studies of childbearing careers in Ghana. First, the study design permits a comparative analysis of fertility among three distinct categories of women: women in a rural setting, indigenous urban women, and a group of urban elite. Previous studies used national data (see Oheneba-Sakyi 1989) and were particularly not useful for the analysis of local-level variation in the timing effect. Second, the data consist of three birth cohorts drawn from births in three historical periods, and therefore it is possible to assess temporal changes in the relationship.

The comparison of urban indigenous, urban elite, and rural women is crucial to our understanding of demographic issues in contemporary Ghana. Over the past two decades, residential and social inequalities have risen steadily in urban areas in Ghana (Songsore and McGranahan 1993). These inequalities mean that the careers of different socioeconomic groups are experienced in increasingly different venues. Thus the use of national aggregated data may be too crude to adequately portray the socioeconomic and personal circumstances that structure the fertility patterns of these different women.

Our results show that the link between the timing of first births and subsequent fertility in Ghana is not as simple as has been perceived. For example, among the 1960s and 1970s birth cohorts in the urban indigenous areas, early childbearing is not linked to subsequent high fertility (because the young teenagers who experience a teenage birth are more likely to be current users of modern contraception after the first birth). In the rural setting in contrast, early childbearing leads to subsequent high fertility for all birth cohorts. In yet another pattern, the urban elite show evidence of delayed childbearing, which translates into subsequent low fertility. Although our analysis is based on data from one country, we believe that our findings may apply to other African countries at similar stages of the fertility transition.

The chapter is organized into four sections. Following the introduction, the theoretical arguments for a linkage between early childbirth and subsequent high fertility are reviewed. This is followed by the description of the study area and the data and methods. The empirical evidence on the timing and subsequent fertility patterns in the five Ghanaian communities are then presented. The chapter concludes with a discussion and conclusion.

PREVIOUS RESEARCH

A relatively well-established finding in the demographic literature is that women who start childbearing early tend to end up having more children. This has been noted in numerous empirical studies, in both developed and developing countries. Several mechanisms have been proposed to account for this relationship. The first mechanism is essentially biological: the earlier a woman has her first birth, the more years of her reproductive span remain after that first birth; and if no attempt is made to limit fertility, the greater duration of reproductive exposure alone will lead to more childbearing (Trussell and Reins 1989). Clearly, the biological explanation depends on an increase in subfecundity and infecundity with increasing age. The ability to reproduce obviously does decline with age, but the age at which the decline begins and the pace of the decline are not known precisely. Most women are infecund by age forty-five, and some studies suggest that fecundity begins to decline sharply in the mid to late 30s (Woods 1994).

The second mechanism involves contraceptive failure. If those women who are younger and older at first birth were to have the same pace of fertility and the same desired family size, women who are younger at first birth will be younger when their preferred family size is reached, and women with an earlier age at first birth will experience more years at risk of an unintended pregnancy assuming comparable patterns of fecundity. The third mechanism is sociological. Early first births can limit the opportunities for young women to pursue activities that might compete with childbearing, and hence early childbearing can foster larger desired family size.

Previous studies of the relationship between the timing of first birth and subsequent fertility in Africa have analyzed the large cross-national surveys conducted under the World Fertility Surveys (WFS) and the Demographic and Health Surveys (DHS) programs. Virtually all studies based on the surveys in these programs have shown a strong association between birth timing and subsequent fertility (Westoff 1992; Oheneba-Sakyi 1989; Kirk and Pillet 1998). Using WFS surveys carried out in 1978–1982 and DHS surveys carried out in 1986–1989, Westoff (1992) analyzes the timing of first birth and subsequent fertility in Africa, and observes a marked association at the national level: countries with high age at first birth tend to have low fertility rates.

Results of the DHS conducted in Ghana since the late 1980s indicate that age at first birth has been rising over the years with a corresponding decline in the total fertility rate (TFR). The median age at first birth reported for women aged 25–49 in the 1988 GDHS was 19.6 This increased to 20.3 for the same age group in the most recent DHS conducted in 1998. Within the same period the TFR declined from 6.4 to 4.6 (Statistical Service of Ghana 1989, 1999). While these national figures are revealing, they do not adequately capture the variation among the different socioeconomic groups and geographic regions. We explore this gap in the empirical sections of this chapter. First, however, we describe the study communities in this research, and the data and methods that the analysis uses.

SOCIAL SETTING

The study was conducted in five communities located in three settlements in Ghana: Accra, Cape Coast, and Otuam (see Fig. 5.1). The three settlements were selected to reflect different levels of socio-economic transformation. Accra is the national capital whereas Cape Coast is the capital of the Central Region. Otuam is located between the two, on the southern coast of Ghana.

Accra. From being a relatively small and homogeneous community, with agriculture and fishing as the mainstay of its economy, Accra has grown into a large heterogeneous metropolis where the informal sector is the main source of employment. Accra today consists of different residential and socioeconomic groups. The Ga (indigenous Accra people), most of whom are in the low socioeconomic class, are concentrated in areas such as Jamestown and Ussher Fort: The higher-status groups can be found in areas such as Airport Residential Area, East Legon, Cantoments, and North Labone. The middle-class areas include Kaneshie and Teshie Nungua. Residents of the high and middle socioeconomic groups are largely first-and second-generation migrants to Accra as well as second generation educated indigenes.

Cape Coast. As the first capital of the then Gold Coast until 1877, Cape Coast enjoyed a period of economic prosperity during the colonial period. The economy of Cape Coast, however, witnessed a significant decline after the transfer of the capital to Accra. In the postindependence period, the growth of Cape Coast has largely been due to its position as a major educational and tourist center. In common with Accra, there exist significant contrasts between the high-class areas of the Ridges and Eyifoa, which house top professional and administrative personnel, and the low-class indigenous areas such as Idan and Brofoyedur, whose residents depend mainly on fishing for their livelihood.

Otuam. Otuam is a small fishing village located in central region about 70 kilometres west of Accra and about 50 kilometres east of Cape Coast. The ethnic composition of the village is predominantly Fante. One distinguishable feature about Otuam is seasonal migration. Residents of the area migrate during the off season to other fishing areas to fish, and may be found at coastal settlements in the central and western regions such as Apam, Mankessim, Mumford, Edina, Abuesi, and Aboadze. Significant developments have occurred in Otuam over the past three or four decades. Educational facilities were established in the early 1950s, following which enrollment rates of children of school-going age increased sharply. A health post was also established in the late 1960s. However, the village still lacks electricity services. From a macroeconomic perspective, the years after 1970 have brought untold hardship to the people. The general economic decline in the country since the 1980s has also affected the township. Poverty has become widespread because of increases in the prices of kerosene and hospital fees, clothes, and food in general. The area used to be a closed forest, but continous tree cutting has left the area with virtually no firewood for cooking. Residents of Otuam therefore have to walk long distances to nearby villages for charcoal and firewood, which are the most common energy sources for cooking.

Within the cities of Accra and Cape Coast a further subdivision was made. From Accra, one elite (Airport) and one indigenous area (Jamestown) were chosen. From the smaller city of Cape Coast, two areas of similar characteristics were studied, namely Ridges/Eyifoa (elite) and Idan (indigenous). Otuam was considered as one geographic unit because of the lack of clearly distinguishable differences in its socioeconomic and residential pattern.

DATA AND METHODS

The analysis presented in this chapter uses data collected during the period July to December 1994, as part of a larger study of fertility change in Accra, Cape Coast, and Otuam. A representative survey was conducted in which 1,200 women were interviewed in the five communities. Three birth cohorts were identified: those born in the 1950s, 1960s, and 1970s. The study focused on women aged 15 to 44 irrespective of their marital status. Since the study was conducted in 1994, women born in the 1950s were aged 35 to 44, those born in the 1960s were aged 25 to 34, and those born in the 1970s were aged 15 to 24. An arbitrary weighted index of 3:2:1 was then chosen to apportion the sample

Fig. 5.1
Southern Ghana Showing the Study Communities

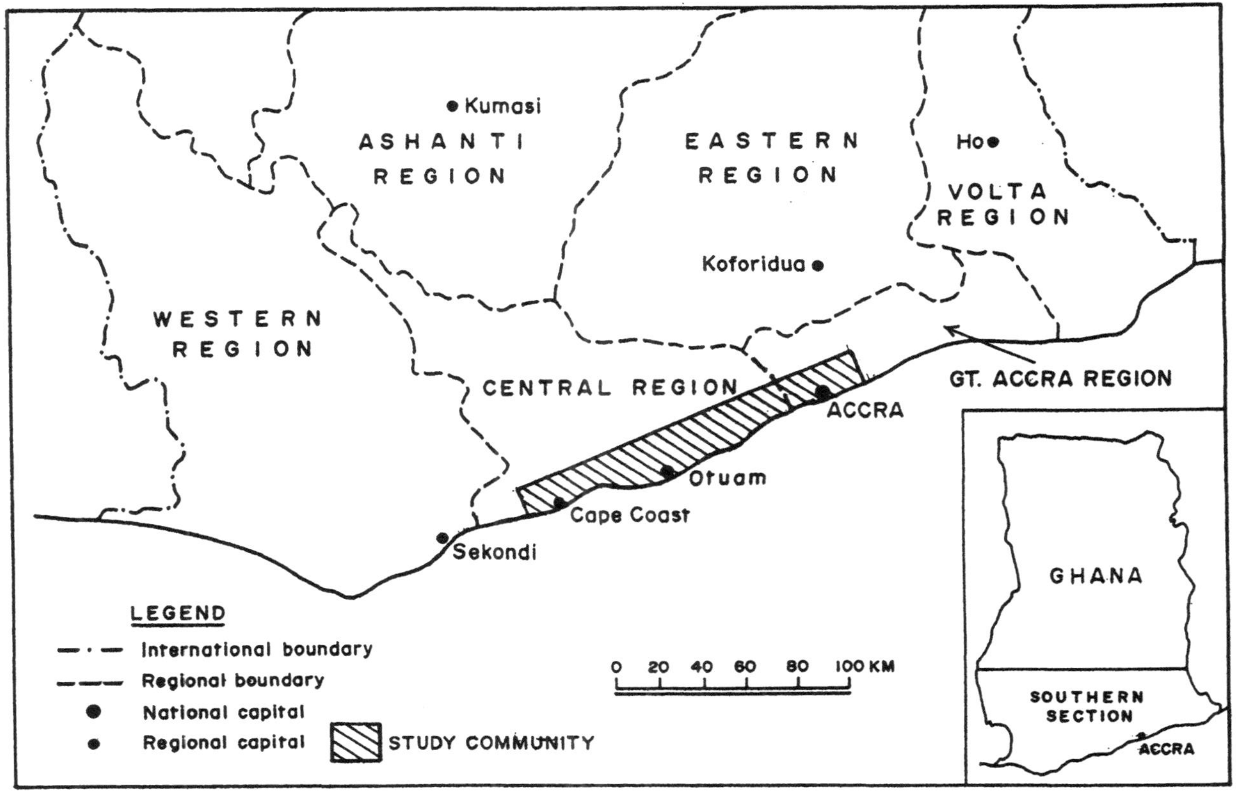

size in relation to the population of the study areas. With the sample size of 1,200, Accra had a sample of 600 women divided equally between Airport and Jamestown; Cape Coast, 400 divided between Ridges/Eyifoa and Idan; and Otuam, 200. For details of the sampling distribution among the study areas see Agyei-Mensah and Aase (1998).

Each cohort has faced its own distinct economic circumstances. By the 1980s, education in Ghana was no longer free, and with the introduction of the economic recovery program in the 1980s, economic opportunities were more strained than was formerly the case. The 1960s birth cohort was born after the country had gained independence from the British in 1957. The massive postindependence drive to establish free educational services and the construction of schools and infrastructure undoubtedly affected the life course patterns of this cohort. The late 1960s and early 1970s also saw increased effort by the government of Ghana to promote family planning. A population policy was established in 1969, followed by the development of a family planning program in the 1970s. These efforts are likely to have influenced birth control usage among the 1960s and 1970s birth cohorts. The 1950s birth cohort, in contrast, was born during a time of relatively low national socioeconomic development. Health services and educational facilities were not well developed and at that time few women were encouraged to attend school (Antwi 1992). If the 1960s was a decade of euphoria and optimism, the 1970s was one of sober reflection. By the middle of the 1970s Ghana had experienced rapid economic decline.

The data collection for this study mainly involved the administration of a structured and an open-ended interview schedule. Besides the interview schedule, information was also collected on community variables such as access to health care, education, the economy, demographic history, and the general way of life. Most of this latter information was obtained through personal observation, interviews, archival material, and published sources.

The interview schedule collected information on the birth histories of women aged 15 to 44, as well as a select set of background characteristics. The fertility histories contain the month and year of each birth, the number of children the woman had ever given birth to, and any experience with child deaths. Cumulative fertility rates were calculated by summing the number of woman years and the number of births to women of that age in the data set. Dividing the number of births by the number of woman years gives an estimate of the number of births per woman. Cumulative births per woman was also calculated for each birth cohort. In the construction of the cumulative fertility curves, the earliest allowed age at maturity is 15 years. All births that occurred prior to age 15 were assumed to occur at age 15.

Errors in the reporting of age and dates of births have plagued fertility surveys conducted in sub-Saharan Africa (see Blanc and Rutenberg 1990). Hence in this study, undoubtedly there are errors resulting from deficiencies in birth and age reporting, especially among the 1950 birth cohorts at Otuam and Idan. However, close inspection of the data indicates that these deficiencies are minimal and do not invalidate the overall pattern of differentials that emerges.

EDUCATIONAL ATTAINMENT

An important socioeconomic variable known to influence the timing of first births is educational attainment. Women with higher education on average delay the onset of childbearing because of the long years spent in school. Higher education also offers literacy and exposure to ideas and values that compete with traditional customs that encourage early childbearing. In this section we examine the educational characteristics of the sampled women, their husbands, and their parents. The data for the women are presented in Table 5.1.

Patterns of female educational attainment are summarized by the percentage of women who have reached certain levels of education: none, primary, middle/JSS, secondary (second)/SSS, tertiary.[1] As expected, the educational background of the women shows significant differences by locality. Women at Airport and the Ridges have relatively higher average educational attainments than women in Jamestown, Idan, and Otuam. There are also cohort differences in educational attainment; with attainment far lower for the 1950s cohorts as compared to the 1960s and the 1970s cohorts. The highest level of women with no schooling is found among the oldest cohort in Otuam with over 90 percent of these women having no education. The comparable figure for this cohort for Idan is about 60 percent and for Jamestown 50 percent.

Education of the husband/partner was also measured (data not shown). The husbands/partners of the women at Airport and the Ridges and Eyifoa have high educational attainments as compared to the husbands in the other study areas. Interestingly, there is a small difference in the percentage of the husbands/partners of the 1950 cohort at Airport and the Ridges who have attained tertiary education. The women in both areas are in relationships with men who have relatively high educational backgrounds.

Finally, indicators of parental backgrounds are also considered (data not shown). Nearly 60 percent of the fathers of the 1950s cohort at Airport had obtained secondary and postsecondary education. Similarly high percentages of the 1950s cohorts at Ridges and Eyifoa have fathers with secondary education or higher. Otuam provides a sharp contrast with virtually all the fathers of the 1950s never having attended school.

Consistent with the pattern found for parental schooling, maternal schooling levels are relatively high for all three birth cohorts in Airport and Ridges. Significant increases across birth cohorts are also evident with mothers of the 1960s and the 1970s cohorts more educated as compared to the mothers of the 1950s cohort. Again Otuam provides a sharp contrast, with the bulk of the mothers having no education. As expected, on average maternal schooling levels are lower than paternal levels (see Agyei-Mensah 1997).

THE TIMING OF FIRST BIRTHS

We examine intercommunity differences in the timing of first births for each of the three cohorts in turn (Tables 5.2, 5.3, and 5.4, respectively).

1950s cohort (Table 5.2). There are intriguing differences among the study areas. Teenage childbearing (births before age 20) is rare among the women at Airport (0.0 percent) and the Ridges and Eyifoa (3.3 percent). In sharp contrast, teenage childbearing is quite common in Otuam (89.2 percent), Idan (85.5 percent), and Jamestown (45.2 percent). Corresponding contrasts are apparent for childbearing after age 20. In the high-class residential areas of Airport and the Ridges and Eyifoa, the bulk of the first births took place at ages 20-24.

Table 5.1
Educational Background of the Women Surveyed By Locality

Area/ Cohort	None	Primary	Middle/ JSS	Second/ SSS	Tertiary	Case
Airport						
1950-59				60% (45)	36% (27)	75
1960-69			4% (3)	48.2% (54)	47.3% (53)	112
1970-79			4.5% (5)	65.5% (74)	34.5% (39)	113
Ridges & Eyifoa						
1950-59		5% (3)	16.7% (10)	71.7% (43)	6.7% (4)	60
1960-69			15.2% (10)	75.8% (50)	9.1% (6)	66
1970-79			10.8% (8)	68.9% (51)	20.3% (15)	74
Jamestown						
1950-59	51.3% (41)	25% (20)	16.3% (13)	7.5% (6)		80
1960-69	7.3% (8)	36.7% (40)	38.5% (42)	16.5% (18)	1.0% (1)	109
1970-79	6.3% (7)	38.7% (43)	43.2% (48)	10.8% (12)	1.0% (1)	111
Idan						
1950-59	59.7% (37)	22.6% (14)	17.7% (11)			62
1960-69	10.6% (7)	30.3% (20)	39.4% (26)	19.7% (13)		66
1970-79	9.7% (7)	58.3% (42)	18.1% (13)	13.9% (10)		72
Otuam						
1959-59	91.1% (51)	5.4% (3)	3.6% (2)			56
1960-69	41.4% (29)	35.7% (25)	22.9% (16)			70
1970-79	37.8% (28)	29.7% (22)	32.4% (24)			74

Similarly in the urban indigenous area of Jamestown most of the women begin childbirth at ages 20 to 24 (47.6 percent) even though an equally high percentage (45.2 percent) begin before age 20.

1960s cohort (Table 5.3). Consistent with the findings for the 1950s cohort, among the 1960s cohort teenage childbearing is uncommon at Airport and the Ridges. However, a different pattern emerges at Jamestown, Idan, and Otuam. Here there has been a sharp decline in the percentage of women giving birth before age 20 as compared to the 1950s cohorts. In Jamestown only 14 percent of the 1960s cohort began childbearing before age 20 as compared to 45 percent among the 1950s cohort. Similarly in Idan, only 24 percent of the 1960s cohort began childbearing before age 20 as compared to 86 percent among the 1950s cohort. The case of Otuam is equally interesting: a very high percentage of the 1960s cohort giving birth before age 20 (69.9 percent) as compared to 89 percent among the 1950s cohort.

Childbearing after age 20 among the 1960s cohort also provides interesting revelations. In the high-class residential area of Airport, the bulk of the first births take place at ages 25 to 29 (50 percent). This contrasts sharply with the situation among the 1950s cohorts where the bulk of the first births occur at ages 20 to 24. The pattern at Ridges and Eyifoa and Jamestown remains the same with the bulk of the first births taking place at ages 20 to 24 as was the case with the 1950s cohorts. The situation at Otuam also remains the same with the bulk of the births occurring before age 20.

The 1970s cohort (Table 5.4). The format of Table 5.4 differs from that of Tables 5.2 and 5.3, with only two age classifications at the entry of motherhood provided, in recognition of the current age of these cohorts: those who began childbearing prior to age 20, and those who started childbearing at age 20 and older. Consistent with the findings for the 1950s and 1960s cohorts, teenage childbearing is uncommon among the 1970s cohort at Airport and the Ridges and Eyifoa. At Airport Residential Area, only 1 percent of the women in this cohort started childbearing before age 20. At the Ridges and Eyifoa, the corresponding percentage is 2.8. These percentages contrast sharply with those of Jamestown (60.4 percent), Idan (73.2 percent), and Otuam (85.2 percent). Thus at Jamestown, Idan, and Otuam, teeenage childbearing is more common among the 1970s cohort than among the 1960s cohort, a finding that runs contrary to a trend toward later entry into childbearing that might have been expected.

Table 5.2
Percentage of First Births before Age 20; 20–24; 25–29; 30+ (1950 Birth Cohorts)

Age	Airport	Ridges	Jamestown	Idan	Otuam
<Age 20	0.0	3.3	45.2	85.5	89.2
Age 20–24	57.2	76.7	47.6	14.5	5.4
Age 25–29	34.6	11.6	1.3	0.0	0.0
Age 30+	3.9	3.4	0.0	0.0	0.0

Table 5.3
Percentage of First Births before Age 20; 20–24; 25–29; 30+ (1960 Birth Cohorts)

Age	Airport	Ridges	Jamestown	Idan	Otuam
<Age 20	0.0	3.0	13.8	24.1	69.9
Age 20–24	26.2	44.0	81.6	74.2	24.3
Age 25–29	50.0	28.7	1.3	1.5	0.0
Age 30+	2.0	6.0	0.0	0.0	0.0

Table 5.4
Percentage of First Births before Age 20; 20–24 (1970 Birth Cohorts)

Age	Airport	Ridges	Jamestown	Idan	Otuam
<Age 20	1.0	2.8	60.4	73.2	85.2
Age 20–24	4.8	8.1	10.1	7.0	1.4

THE PACE OF SUBSEQUENT FERTILITY

Figure 5.2 shows the cumulative number of births for the 1950s cohorts in the five study areas. There exist substantial variations in cumulative births among the study areas, with the lowest reported by women from Airport and the Ridges and the highest at Idan and Otuam. Thus by age 44 years, women at Idan and Otuam had given birth to about 7 and 8 children, respectively, compared to 3 for those in Airport, 4 for the Ridges and Eyifoa, and 5 for Jamestown.

Fig. 5.2
Cumulative Number of Births of 1950s Birth Cohorts by Area of Residence

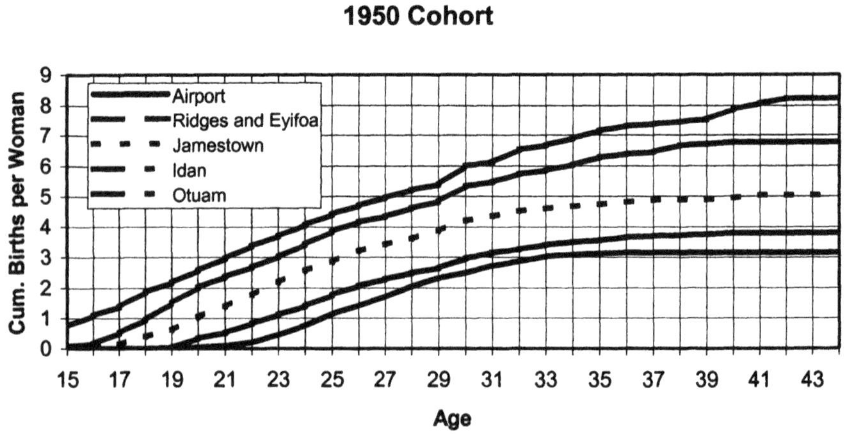

Source: Agyei-Mensah and Aase (1998).

Figure 5.3 shows the cumulative number of births for the 1960s cohort. Note that the curves for Jamestown, the Ridges, and Airport nearly overlap. This is an indication that completed fertility is not high in Jamestown despite the relatively high rate of teenage births. At age thirty-four the cumulative number of births for the 1960s birth cohort in Jamestown (2.4) is almost on par with that of Airport (2.1) and Ridges (2.3). Another interesting finding is the small difference between Airport and the Ridges in the cumulative number of births for the 1960s cohorts. In contrast to the 1950s cohort, for which there is a marked difference between these two areas in cumulative fertility patterns, there is little difference between the areas for this cohort.

Fig. 5.3
Cumulative Number of Births of 1960s Birth Cohorts by Locality and Residence

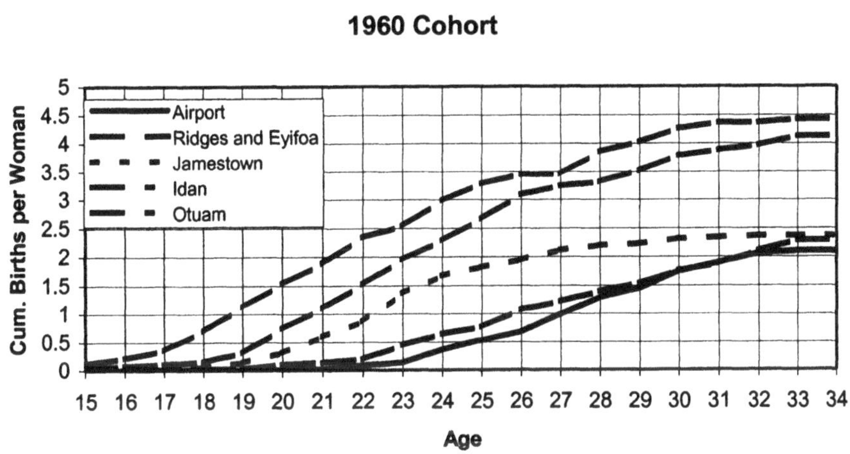

Fig. 5.4
Cumulative Number of Births of 1970s Cohorts by Locality and Residence

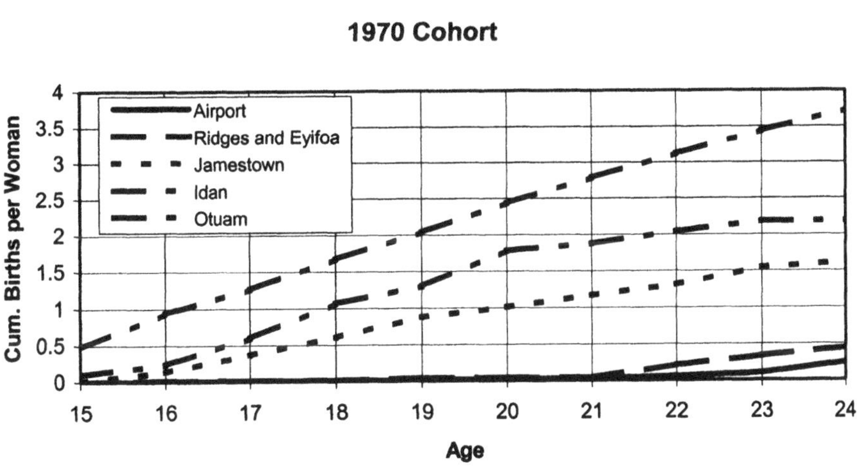

The 1970s birth cohort is yet to reach the reproductive peak. From their cumulative fertility to date, however, it is possible to get a good feeling for their likely final completed fertility (see Fig. 5.4). Three general patterns emerge. The first is the high fertility among women at Otuam. The second is the relatively low fertility of 1.6 children among women at Jamestown. The third is the very low fertility among women at the Airport Residential Area and the Ridges and Eyifoa.

DISCUSSION

The results of the analysis demonstrate that both the timing of births and cumulative fertility differ according to social setting and birth cohort.

The 1950s Birth Cohorts

The variations in birth timing and subsequent fertility that can be observed among the 1950s birth cohorts can be explained in part by differences in educational attainments and in part by differences in family backgrounds and societal context. As discussed above, the 1950s cohort at Airport is more educated as compared to the same cohort in other areas. The long period spent in school might itself be a factor in delaying the onset of childbearing.

The relatively high educational levels of these women should also make them more receptive to new innovations, ideas, and alternative lifestyles that are compatible with delays in birth timing and small family sizes. It is interesting to note that among the 1950s cohort at Airport, the ideal family size is about 3.4 children whereas their cumulative number of births as well as the mean number of children ever born is also 3.2. Thus their fertility desires are rather close on average to actual fertility levels, suggesting that these women make a deliberate effort to attain their fertility desires. One might infer that the idea of family limitation exists in this group. Note that the mean for Ghana as a whole, according to the Ghana DHS, was 5.5 in 1993, 4.4 in 1993, and 4.3 in 1998 (Statistical Service of Ghana 1999). The relatively low cumulative fertility is also indicative of improvements in health and child survival rates, which make the women more confident that their children will survive. The figures also imply that women adopt birth control to stop having additional children once they achieve their desired family size goals. This in turn could be a response to the recent economic adversity, which has reinforced the desire for quality of children instead of quantity.

Compared to the elite areas of Airport and Ridges, the 1950s birth cohort at Jamestown begin childbearing relatively early: about 45 percent of these women begin childbearing before age twenty. Cumulative fertility is also high. We explain this as a response to their background characteristics as well as societal factors. Let us begin with evidence regarding their educational backgrounds. Fifty-one percent of the 1950s cohort at Jamestown did not attend school, only about 25 percent had obtained primary education, and none had attained tertiary education. Some facet of the broader societal changes within Accra should be noted here. Robertson (1984) writes that the interwar period marked the first substantial changes in the social and economic conditions of women in Accra. In Accra, until after World War II it was not common to send girls to school. These developments did not automatically alter the class structure in Accra, but did contribute to modest improvement in educational levels of women in the traditional Ga enclaves. Thus the 1950s cohort can be regarded as the generation that began to be affected by the benefits of education.

The high number of teenage births and the resultant high fertility among the 1950s cohort at Idan and Otuam can also be explained by their backgrounds as well as structural factors. Many of the 1950s cohort at Idan and Otuam never attended school (nearly 60 percent and 91 percent in Idan and Otuam, respectively). Children are valued for the household chores they provide, and as a major source of old-age security. The case of Idan is particularly interesting, considering the fact that Cape Coast was the first capital of colonial Ghana and its population had an early lead in school attainment. This suggests that, despite the existence of schools in the area, the majority of local people in fishing suburbs such as Idan did not send their children to school, probably because they were needed to assist in the fishing industry, or because the parents saw little return to schooling.

In contrast to Idan, the explanation for Otuam is more structural. The women begin childbearing early because school-going was not a novelty at the time. For example, no school facilities existed in the area until the early 1950s, when an elementary school was established. The 1960 census of Ghana records gave the overall illiteracy rate for Otuam as 85.2 percent and 95.2 percent for women in the area aged 15+ (Agyei-Mensah 1997). Because there were few occupations that allowed women to be self-supporting, it was in their best interest to start childbearing early. The early ages at first birth resulted in longer periods of exposure to unplanned births, thus contributing to high fertility. Early ages at first birth also forclosed opportunities for academic or occupational achievement. The high teenage birth rate also finds a rational explanation in a system in which marriage and family formation are important social norms and are major mechanisms for maintaining social systems. Part of the explanation for this probably lies in the cultural factors that necessitate the demand for a high number of children. Perhaps women of this era adhered to the increasing pressures of the pevailing social norms of domesticity and early parenting. Children did not present an opportunity cost to women because they were mainly involved in the fishing industry and their children could accompany them to work. It is also possible that some of the 1950s cohort at Otuam decided to have large families with considerations of their old age in mind.

The 1960s Birth Cohorts

The relatively higher social development at Airport and the Ridges and Eyifoa also applies to the 1960s cohort. About 47 percent of the 1960s cohort at Airport attained tertiary education as compared to 36 percent among the 1950s cohort. These relatively well-educated women also tend to marry men with higher educational backgrounds. The relatively high educational backgrounds of the 1960s cohort makes it more likely that they know and practice birth control, especially in the case of the unmarried, but also, that they space and postpone births on the part of those who are married.

More macrolevel factors may have also played a role. The accelerated development plan introduced by the government of Nkrumah in 1951, and implemented in 1952, as well as the Educational Act of 1961 provided for the rapid development of education at all levels. The implementation of these plans produced quantitative progress in the development of education in the country (Antwi 1992). These developments contributed to the situation where the 1960s cohort is more likely than the 1950s cohort to have progressed to high educational levels. Progress in medicine in Ghana in general has also meant a considerably greater life expectancy, and also the risks associated with pregnancy and birth have been significantly reduced. The introduction of population and family planning programs since the late 1960s and early 1970s has also meant that increasing segments of the population have access to family planning methods.

The situation with respect to the 1960s cohort at Jamestown is somewhat different. As already noted, the educational levels of these women are much lower than in Airport and the Ridges. But we should also note that despite these differences there has been a significant improvement in educational levels in Jamestown. We suspect that these improvements may have contributed to the relatively low rate of teenage births recorded among the 1960s cohort in Jamestown. Their cumulative fertility curve in Fig. 5.3, puzzling at first sight, calls for an understanding of socioeconomic changes within the broader society. Developments in education and industry in Accra after independence in 1957 greatly affected the socioeconomic fortunes of the 1960s cohort. Unlike the 1950s cohort, most of these women in Jamestown received some form of education. Increased educational opportunities pushed the women outside the mainstream fishing activity. Thus there was a gradual shift in their occupational structures away from the traditional fishing industry into the cash economy, among other things trading in imported goods made available by industrial policies (Robertson 1984; Clark 1994).

With increased education and the rise in service sector opportunities, women in Jamestown began to control substantial amounts of cash leading to economic independence from men. This trend was accentuated by the economic crisis in the 1970s and diminishing fish catches, both of which diminished the economic fortunes of men. As a consequence of the shrinking economic opportunity for men, there has been growing infidelity, broken marriages, female-headed households, and a relatively large number of unmarried women (Songsore and McGranahan 1996). If we examine more closely the marriage profile of these women, especially the percentage unmarried, further important differences appear. In the 1960s cohort, women at Jamestown have the highest percentage of the unmarried. A little over 18 percent of these women have never been married, as compared to 17 percent at Airport, 15 percent at Ridges, 4.3 at

Otuam, and 1.5 percent at Idan. It is some of these changes that have affected reproductive behavior leading to the apparent low cumulative fertility observed.

Why do we not observe a similar pattern for Idan in Cape Coast? Our explanation is that the socioeconomic changes were different. Most of the women in Jamestown were able to enter into trading because of the buoyant trading activity in Accra. In contrast, Cape Coast was a relatively deprived economy heavily dominated by the traditional fishing industry. Even though there were some improvements with the introduction of the outboard motor in 1959 and the nylon sieve net in 1967, these changes in the fishing industry were not accompanied by any substantial occupational specialization. Technological change took place within the existing traditional framework and did not require any radical alteration in technological know-how (Hinderink and Sterkenburg 1975). Thus trading activities were not as buoyant as at Accra. Poverty was also more acute in Cape Coast, and women are less autonomous than the women in Jamestown, a situation that made the women more dependent on men and gave them less control over their own fertility. Educational backgrounds also differed markedly between the 1960s cohort at Jamestown and Idan.

The 1970s Birth Cohorts

As was the case with the 1960s birth cohort in the elite areas of Airport, the Ridges, and Eyifoa, the 1970s cohort also have well-educated parents, which means that these women come from a more affluent class, by virtue of their educational status. Hence the social and economic fortunes of these women were far less affected by the severe economic crisis that hit the country at the end of the 1970s. Teenage childbearing is uncommon among these women. We see this development as a manifestation of ideational changes among this particular cohort. In pieces that have appeared recently in the fertility literature, Bongaarts and Watkins (1996) and Montgomery and Casterline (1998) have advanced a social interaction model to account for changes in the prevalence of fertility control. Even though these mechanisms are likely to differ from one society to another, we strongly believe that among the Ghanaian elite rising Westernization and exposure to the outside world has fostered a culture that is incompatible with early fertility. Their values with regard to childbearing have been shaped by the socialization process through contact with the immediate family, friends, and neighbors, as well as the communities within which they reside. Exposure to the outside world through modernizing media and communication and traveling has also contributed.

One way of gauging the extent of ideational change among these cohorts is by looking at their fertility preferences and their gender role attitudes. It is instructive to note that the 1970 cohorts in the elite areas tend to have relatively low family size ideals especially in comparison to the 1950 cohorts. For example, at Airport, whereas 53 percent of the 1970s cohort preferred two children, only 20 percent of the 1950s cohort at Airport preferred two children. In addition, whereas only 5 percent of the 1970s cohort at Airport preferred four children, 48 percent of the 1950s cohort wanted that many.

We can also detect a clear change with respect to gender-role attitudes. For example, the more recent birth cohorts (1970s cohort) were more in favor of men cooking than the 1950s cohort. Ninety-two percent of the 1970s cohort at Airport approve of men cooking, whereas only 56 percent of the 1950s cohort approve of men cooking. With regard to why men should assist in cooking, a substantial fraction of the 1970s cohort at Airport tend to see cooking as a duty to be shared by both men and women, as evidenced by the relatively high percentage of the women who gave responses such as equality and shared responsibility. In contrast, not much has changed with respect to gender role attitudes among the 1970s cohort at Jamestown, Idan, and Otuam. This shows that social change does not necessarily lead to changes in traditional attitudes and values.

Value changes among the elites of Airport became clear to us during an interview with two female students resident at Airport. Abena, a student in her twenties, had lived at Airport since she was twelve. Asked about her plans for the future and her goals and aspirations, she replied:

> These days jobs are hard to come by. The men are also not available. Most women therefore prefer to work for some time to earn some income and buy some basic things before settling down. Others have opted to broaden their horizons by embarking on professional studies or by taking postgraduate courses at the universities, while others have traveled abroad to pursue further studies.

Akua, a twenty-two-year-old student also resident at Airport, had this to say on the issue of gender-role-based responsibility for household activities such as cooking. She indicated:

> Times have changed. With modernization, women are pursuing careers. Because of this, women's roles have changed and responsibilities in the home have to be shared.

Akua went on to tell us about her background.

> I was born in 1972 at Mamprobi, a suburb of Accra. When I was eleven years old, my parents moved to Airport Residential Area. My father has university education and is a journalist by profession, and my mother is a teacher. I am the only child of my parents, and am currently a second-year undergraduate student at the University.

Akua feels that the ideal number of children that a couple should have is two. According to her, this number enables a couple to take very good care of the children and provide them with the foundation they need to progress in life. She has a boyfriend and started using contraceptives at age twenty-one. She wants to get married at age twenty-six, by which time she hopes to have finished her master's degree. According to Akua:

> I want to get married at that age, because I want to get a sound education and self-satisfaction in life and also be part of the elite in society. It is through higher education that I can reach my goals and aspirations in life. I want to contribute to the support of my

family, and I also want security for the future, so that I will not be a burden on my children when I grow old and can no longer work. In case I find myself in a government job, then I will depend on social security or pension. Aside from this I want to have some investments as well as income-generating ventures.

The wish to pursue a career and postpone marriage appears to be important among women within an environment that promotes higher education and higher aspiration as pertains in the Airport and Ridges residential areas. These young women with their plans for advanced education and their career aspirations delay forming any type of union, and are particularly unlikely to become pregnant while unmarried and to have a child. Increased knowledge about and access to contraceptive services have also given them more options for controlling the timing of their fertility. And it is likely that a significant number of those who do get pregnant would resort to abortions (see also Caldwell et al. 1992 on signs of demographic change in Nigeria). Besides their own value orientations, the influence of their parents goes a long way toward shaping their reproductive outcomes.

The picture that emerges from the elite areas of Airport, the Ridges, and Eyifoa is not what we find in the urban indigenous areas of Jamestown and Idan and in the rural area of Otuam. In these areas, most of the first births take place before age twenty. Thus teenage childbearing is very common. Conversations with some of the women in Jamestown and Idan reveals that many of the first births were unplanned and occurred outside marriage. The women did not use or insist on effective contraception from their partners prior to the birth of the first child. The problem here is not lack of education. Indeed only 6 percent of the 1970s cohort at Jamestown have not been to school, and in Idan the figure is 10 percent. We believe the relatively high number of teenage births among these women has to do with macrolevel changes, especially economic crisis in recent years and the breakdown in social and moral attitudes among the youth. Long-established cultural norms that discouraged births outside of marriage are no longer taken seriously. A teenage mother without a husband is no longer seen as something strange, but is gradually being accepted as a way of life. Compounding this, recent economic hardships have put tremendous pressure on families, with most families unable to provide the necessary economic support for their children. This has led to a situation where many of these young women resort to sexual liaisons with elderly men for money.

Even though their counterparts in the elite areas have also been made vulnerable by recent economic hardships, the pressure for cash and other items will be higher among women from poorer family backgrounds such as those living in Jamestown, Idan, and Otuam. In addition, the drive for higher academic laurels and career achievement is not so strong among this group as compared to those in the elite areas. Interviews with a sample of the women also revealed that many of their parents are unable to provide them with their entertainment needs. As a result, some of these women go out frequently in search of fulfilling leisure time. For these various reasons, the risk of pregnancy and childbirth is higher among adolescents in urban indigenous and rural areas as compared to those in the elite areas.

What is remarkable about the relatively high rate of teenage births in Jamestown in particular is that these are not followed by high cumulative fertility later in the reproductive career. This remarkable finding has also been observed in a recent study in rural South Africa (see Garenne et al. 2000). We attribute this change to a rationalization of sexual behavior after the initial first births. Even though sexual activity may continue after the first child is born, the young women tend to adopt more efficient contraceptives and take up a trade or reenter school. These are decisions that are incompatible with caring for an additional child. Also, given the gradual breakup of the extended family system in urban settings, support from kin is not likely to be forthcoming. We shoud also note here that many adolescents in Ghana shy away from family planning clinics prior to the birth of the first child. Only once they have been pregnant do they resort to these clinics. The recourse to family planning clinics after the first birth might also explain why the early births are not followed by subsequent high fertility (see also Garenne et al. 2000).

Finally, the high number of teenage births and the subsequent high cumulative fertility among the 1970s cohort of Otuam could be attributed to socio-cultural forces. As a rural area along the coast and away from the main Accra-Cape Coast road, the town continues to follow the tradition of early and high fertility as a social status symbol.

CONCLUSIONS

This chapter examines the relationship between the timing of first births and subsequent fertility in five communities and three birth cohorts in southern Ghana. Substantial differences in the timing and pace of subsequent fertility emerged from the study. In particular, we have identified three patterns: early childbearing and subsequent low fertility, delayed childbearing and subsequent low fertility, and early childbearing and subsequent high fertility.

Although the findings of the study support the view that women who start childbearing early tend to have more children, as seen, for example, in the case of the rural area of Otuam, they also challenge the assumption that early childbearing necessarily leads to subsequent high fertility. In the case of the 1960s and 1970s cohorts at Jamestown, early childbearing did not lead to subsequent high fertility. Although women in the elite areas of Airport, the Ridges, and Eyifoa come from a more affluent class by virtue of their educational statuses and family background, their reproductive behavior suggests a conscious appreciation of the importance of birth timing and the preparedness to delay births in pursuance of higher education and career aspirations in the future. Thus apart from their educational backgrounds, there is an ideational element that influences their reproductive behavior. One should also not lose sight of recent economic hardships that have led to quality-quantity tradeoffs in reproductive decision making.

The results of the study have important theoretical and practical policy implications for sub-Saharan African countries. With respect to theoretical issues, the study shows that an early childbirth does not necessarily signal a subsequent high fertility. Indeed, an early unplanned birth can lead to the adoption of more effective modern contraceptives in an environment where the extended family is crumbling and social support systems are inadequate.

In the last two decades, nationally representative data on fertility, health, and living standards have been collected in Ghana. However, the results from these surveys are presented at the aggregate level and do not permit much geographic disaggregation. By situating the research at the local level, we have been able to delineate some of the varied social settings and communities that matter beyond the national level. It is hoped that by demonstrating the importance of social setting and local community, we will encourage those interested in the study of the African fertility transition to give more attention to local-level variations in the phenomenon.

NOTES

This chapter builds upon the doctoral dissertation of Samuel Agyei-Mensah presented to the Norwegian University of Science and Technology, and supervised by Asbjorn Aase. Funding for this study was provided by the Norwegian Research Council (NFR) and the Nordic African Institute (Uppsala, Sweden). The authors are grateful to John B. Casterline for comments made on the chapter.

1. At one time, the educational structure was based on 17 years of preuniversity schooling (6 years primary, 4 years middle, 5 years secondary, and 2 years sixth form). This has now been reduced to 12 years. The new structure consists of 6 years of primary, 3 years of junior secondary school (JSS), and 3 years of senior secondary school (SSS).

REFERENCES

Agyei-Mensah, S. (1997). *Fertility Change in a Time and Space Perspective: Lessons from Three Ghanaian Settlements.* Doctoral Dissertation. Norwegian University of Science and Technology, 361 pages.

Agyei-Mensah, S., and A. Aase. (1998). Patterns of fertility change in Ghana: A time and space perspective. *Geografiska Annaler* 80B(4): 101–113.

Althaus, S.F. (1991). Early marriage and childbearing remain common in much of the developing world even as fertility falls. *International Family Planning Perspectives* 17(3): 119–120.

Antwi, M.K. (1992). *Education, Society and Development in Ghana.* Unimax Publishers Limited.

Blanc, A.K., and N. Rutenberg. (1990). Assessment of the quality of data on age at first sexual intercourse, age at first marriage, and age at first birth in the Demographic and Health Surveys. In *An Assessment of DHS-I Data Quality, DHS Methodological Reports*, No.1. Columbia, MD: Institute for Resource Development.

Bongaarts, J., and S. Watkins. (1996). Social interactions and contemporary fertility transitions. *Population and Development Review* 22: 639–682.

Caldwell, J.C., I. Oruboloye, and P. Caldwell. (1992). Fertility decline in Africa: A new type of transition? *Population and Development Review*, pp. 211–242.

Clark, G. (1994). *Onions Are My Husband: Survival and Accumulation by West Africa Market Women*. Chicago: The University of Chicago Press.

Davis, K., and J. Blake. (1956). Social structure and fertility: an analytical framework. *Economic Development and Cultural Change* 4: 211–235.

Garenne, M., S. Tollman, and K. Kahn. (2000). Premarital fertility in rural South Africa: A challenge to existing population policy. *Studies in Family Planning* 31(1): 47–54.

Hinderink, J., and J. Sterkenburg. (1975). *Anatomy of an African Town: A Socio-economic Study of Cape Coast, Ghana*. Utrecht, The Netherlands: Department of Geography, University of Utrecht.

Kirk, D., and B. Pillet. (1998). Fertility levels, trends, and differentials in sub-Saharan Africa in the 1980s and 1990s. *Studies in Family Planning* 29(1): 1–22.

Montgomery, M.R., and J.B. Casterline. (1996). Social learning, social Influence, and new models of fertility. In J.B. Casterline and R. Lee (eds.). Fertility in the United States: new patterns new theories. *Population and Development Review*, 22, Supplement, pp. 151–175.

Morgan, S.P., and R.R. Rindfuss. (1999). Re-examining the link of early childbearing to marriage and to subsequent fertility. *Demography* 36(1): 59–75.

Oheneba-Sakyi, Y. (1989). Cohort shifts in the timing of births in Ghana. *Sociological Perspectivs* 32(4): 485–500.

Robertson, C. (1984). *Sharing the Same Bowl: A Socioeconomic History of Women and Class in Accra, Ghana*. Ann Arbor: University of Michigan Press.

Songsore, J., and G. McGranahan. (1993). Environment, wealth and health: towards an analysis of intra-urban differentials within the Greater Accra Metropolitan Area, Ghana. *Environment and Urbanization* 5(2): 10–34.

Songsore, J., and M. McGranahan. (1996). *Women and Household Environmental Care in the Greater Accra Metropolitan Area, Ghana*. Urban Environmental Series, Report No. 2. Stockholm Environmental Institute.

Statistical Service of Ghana (1989). *Ghana Demographic and Health Survey 1988*.

Statistical Service of Ghana (1999). *Ghana Demographic and Health Survey 1998*.

Trussell, J., and J. Menken. (1978). Early childbearing and subsequent fertility. *Family Planning Perspectives* 10: 209–218.

Trussell, J., and K.I. Reins. (1989). Age at first marriage and age at first birth. *United Nations Population Bulletin*, ST/ESA/Series N/26, New York, 1989.

Westoff, C. (1992). *Age at Marriage, Age at First birth, and Fertility in Africa*. World Bank Technical Paper No 169. Washington, DC: World Bank.

Woods, J.W. (1994). *Dynamics of Human Reproduction: Biology, Biometry and Demography*. New York: Aldine de Gruyter.

6

CHANGES IN REPRODUCTIVE IDEOLOGY AND ITS CONTROL FROM NATURAL TO LIMITED FERTILITY REGIMES IN MALAWI

Eliya Msiyaphazi Zulu and Ezekiel Kalipeni

INTRODUCTION

There has been an increased interest in the role of men in making reproductive decisions, particularly concerning use of modern contraceptives and family limitation. This interest has been fueled by the empirical studies conducted to understand factors affecting contraceptive use and unmet need for family planning, which have demonstrated that men's opposition is one of the most important causes of unmet need for family planning among women (Yinger 1998; Casterline et al. 1997; Biddlecom et al. 1997; Bankole and Singh 1998; Westoff and Bankole 1998). However, what is not clear is whether men's opposition reflects their desire to have more children, as had been argued by other studies (e.g., Ezeh 1993; Bankole 1995; Omondi-Odhiambo 1997; Dodoo 1998), or a reaction to their exclusion from family planning programs. When modern contraceptives were introduced in sub-Saharan Africa they were targeted at women in the childbearing ages, with no attention paid to men. The focus on women was warranted not only because most of the contraceptives were female based, but because the services were delivered through the existing maternal and child health programs, which are predominantly patronized by women (Watkins and Hodgson 1998; Watkins 1993; Becker 1996). Additionally, it was argued that African men were less inclined to limit their families than women because women bear the biological burdens associated with frequent childbearing, and operate in a sociocultural and economic environment that make high fertility beneficial for both men and women but places childrearing costs primarily on women (Caldwell 1977). The dominance of men in making reproductive decisions has been considered one of the key features of African culture that sustained the region's high fertility (Caldwell and Caldwell 1987). However, men's readiness to support their wives' use of contraception when they are specifically targeted by programs (Drennan 1998; Roudi and Ashford 1996) shows the need to be cautious about accepting too readily the notion that African men oppose family planning because they stand to benefit more from high fertility than African women.

A major weakness in demographic research in general, and in studying the role of men in reproductive decisions in sub-Saharan Africa in particular, has been the tendency to ignore the historical and cultural context of the African reproductive regime [see Mbacke (1994) for similar sentiments]. The immense interest and concern to enable couples in developing countries to control their fertility has propelled researchers and programs to focus on modern methods of family planning because of their effectiveness in averting unplanned childbearing. However, modern methods of contraception were introduced in societies with existing reproductive beliefs and practices that, if well understood, could improve our understanding of how people perceive and comprehend modern family planning.

Using data gained from localized studies, this chapter examines the relative role of men, women, and other people in making reproductive decisions regarding use of traditional and modern methods of family planning in Malawi. Specifically, the chapter examines the rationale for men's feeble support of modern contraception by comparing their decision-making role in relation to traditional versus modern methods. Understanding the sociocultural context in which traditional methods are used, how users of the methods are determined, and who plays key decision-making roles may enhance our understanding of the confluence of gender relations and reproductive control in sub-Saharan Africa.

DATA AND CONTEXT

This study utilizes qualitative and quantitative data collected in three rural and two urban areas in Malawi. The quantitative data are drawn from a survey on Traditional Methods of Child Spacing in Malawi (TMCSM), which was conducted in 1988 in three culturally divergent rural districts (Rumphi, Mchinji, and Chiradzulu) (Srivastava and M'manga 1991). These data are used to measure the relative influence of wives, husbands, and other people in making decisions relating to use of modern and traditional methods of family planning, using multinomial logistic regression. Although these data appear relatively old for examining current gender roles in reproductive decision making in Malawi, they are valuable since the issues being addressed are pertinent to many settings in sub-Saharan Africa (including Malawi) where use of traditional methods of family planning is still prominent.

In order to understand the sociocultural context in which various reproductive beliefs and practices are formulated and played out, a qualitative study (using focus group discussions and in-depth interviews) was organized in the rural areas covered by the 1988 TMCSM survey between September 1994 and January 1995. The qualitative interviews were organized to capture experiences of men and women at different stages of their reproductive spans. Young men and women with one to three children represented people at the beginning of their reproductive period; middle-aged men and women with four to five children represented those in the middle of their reproductive span; while old men and women with 6 or more children represented those approaching the end of their reproductive period. In total, twenty-two focus group discussions and sixty in-depth interviews were conducted. These data provide more insights into the relative roles of husbands, wives, and other people (particularly the elderly) in making decisions regarding use of modern and traditional methods of family planning. The qualitative data were analyzed using Nud*ist (qualitative software), and the quotes presented in this chapter are reflective of what was said across the groups. Wherever excerpts from more than one focus group participant are used, the different participants are distinguished by "m#" for men and "f#" for women.

The three study sites differ substantially with respect to various social and cultural measures, as shown in Table 6.1. Rumphi has a strict patrilineal lineage and kinship system, whereby marriage involves much higher levels of bride price than the other areas, and there is also a higher incidence of polygamy. Chiradzulu has a strict matrilineal system of lineage and kinship where no bride price is paid by the man's side when getting married. The two ethnic groups interviewed in Mchinji follow mixed systems of lineage. Although the Chewas are traditionally matrilineal, they mostly follow patrilocal residence and pay a limited amount of bride price. The Ngonis of Mchinji, who are patrilineal and follow patrilocal residence, pay a sizable amount of bride price, though much less than what is paid in Rumphi. However, the two groups are combined in this study because their marriage and kinship systems have increasingly become similar as they have shared space, speak the same language, and have intermarried over the years. Mchinji had the highest levels of both fertility and mortality, while Rumphi has the lowest mortality and Chiradzulu the lowest fertility. The three regions also differ with regard to the level of urbanization and the population's level of education. The northern region is the least urbanized and structurally developed of the three regions, although the region has much higher levels of literacy and child survival than the other two regions. The TMCSM data showed that of the currently married women who were susceptible to become pregnant 6.0, 4.7, and 0.6 percent were using a modern contraceptive in Chiradzulu, Rumphi, and Mchinji, respectively. Contraceptive use has increased remarkably in the three areas as demonstrated by the 1998 Malawi Diffusion and Ideation Change Study (Miller et al. 2001) whereby 16.4 and 22.4 percent of the currently married women were using modern methods in Rumphi and Mchinji, respectively, and 8.4 percent were using traditional methods in both sites. At the national level, the percentage of married women using modern contraceptives increased from 7 percent to 12 percent between 1992 and 1996, while those using traditional methods remained constant at 6 percent (Malawi Government 1997).

Table 6.1
Social and Demographic Characteristics of Study Sites

	REGION		
Characteristic	South	Central	North
Ethnic Composition	Lomwes/ Yaos	Ngonis/ Chewas	Tumbukas
District/Area	Chiradzulu/ Balaka	Mchinji	Rumphi
Total Fertility Rate	5.9	8.4	6.7
Infant Mortality Rate[a]	162	185	137
Contraceptive Prevalence Rates			
Modern Methods 1988	6.0%	0.6%	4.7%
Modern Methods 1998	12.5%	22.4%	16.4%
Traditional Methods 1998	2.8%	8.3%	8.4%
Women Without Formal Schooling			
1988	54.6%	39.9%	5.6%
1998	62.7%	38.2%	4.3%
Men Without Formal Schooling			
1988	21.1%	19.1%	4.8%
1998	42.2%	19.0%	3.1%
Women in Polygamous Unions			
1988	16.1%	14.0%	26.7%
1998	19.8%	23.5%	28.5%
Religion (1998)			
Catholic	15.8%	23.4%	15.0%
Protestant	18.0%	73.1%	83.6%
Moslem	63.9%	0.2%	1.2%
Other	2.3%	3.3%	0.2%
Kinship System	Matrilineal	Mixed	Patrilineal
Bride Wealth[b]	Nothing	K100	K1000
Residence	Matrilocal	Mixed	Patrilocal
Rights Over Children	Mother	Mixed	Father
Inheritance of land	Daughters	Mixed	Sons
Number of Cases			
Women	273	550	288
Men	70	432	292

Note:
[a] The infant mortality rates refer to the whole district (and based on census data).
[b] Malawi's currency is called Kwacha (K), and the exchange rate to the USA dollar as of January 1997 was about K15 to $1.
Source: Zulu, 2001.

RESULTS

Initiators of Decisions to Use Traditional and Modern Methods of Family Planning

TMCSM respondents who had ever used traditional contraceptive strings, oral medicines, or modern methods of family planning were asked to specify whoinitiated the decision to use the method. Interviewers were asked to insist on knowing the person who initiated the decision. The obvious limitation of this categorization is that it did not make provision for cases where the decision was made jointly or mutually. Additionally, decisions to use contraceptives evolve over time, and people usually make such decisions after consulting with a series of other people with whom they socialize (Rosenfield et al. 1973).

Contraceptive strings are made from barks of certain trees, and are worn around the woman's waist throughout the time when a conception is not desired. Oral traditional medicines are taken in liquid form, either in the morning after intercourse or immediately after or before having intercourse. Oral medicines are believed to prevent conception by rendering the man's semen powerless. Respondents who had ever used the strings or the oral medicines were asked to specify the person who initiated the decision to use the method. Respondents who were currently using any modern method were also asked to specify who initiated the decision to use the method. Answers to the question were precoded into the following four categories: (1) yourself, (2) husband/wife, (3) mother/grandmother, and (4) others. The last two categories have been combined in the analysis because there were very few cases in the "other" category, and most of those who specified this category indicated that the initiator was an elderly woman.

The percentage distributions of respondents who initiated decisions to use the three types of methods are presented in Table 6.2. The results show marked differences in the levels of use of the two traditional methods; more people in Rumphi than in Mchinji and Chiradzulu districts used oral medicines, while more people in Mchinji than in Rumphi and Chiradzulu used traditional contraceptive strings. Although the regional comparisons in the proportion of decisions initiated by the three groups of initiators are somewhat compromised by the small number of users in the TMCSM survey, the patterns demonstrate striking differences between men's and women's reports on the relative role of wives, husbands, and other people in initiating decisions relating to use of modern versus traditional methods.

The results show that at least two-thirds (64 percent for strings and 67 percent for oral medicines) of all decisions relating to use of traditional methods are initiated by a member of the conjugal family (either the wife or the husband). Additionally, wives play a greater role in initiating use of traditional methods than other people and men, in that order. Although both men and women underscore the importance of the conjugal couple in initiating these decisions, men's reports tend to demonstrate higher levels of other people's role than women's reports. For instance, while 31 and 22 percent of women reported that decisions to use strings and oral medicines were made by other people, respectively, 41 and 44 percent of men reported such decisions to have been initiated by this group.

These patterns suggest that men generally think that their wives do not play a prominent role in decision making about use of traditional methods; that is, if husbands did not initiate decisions to use the methods, they think the decisions were initiated by other people, rather than their wives. The discrepancy between men and women's reports are even greater for oral medicines where women report that 62 percent of the decisions were initiated by wives, while men reported that 29 percent of the decisions were initiated by wives. This is not surprising since oral medicines are drunk by women; it is therefore conceivable that the woman would decide to use the medicines even without the husband knowing, and if he knows, for her to give him the impression that the decision was initiated by the elderly members of the extended family.

When it comes to modern methods, there is a substantial shift in the relative role of wives, husbands, and other people in initiating use of contraception. The major shift relates to husbands, who are responsible for initiating 56 percent of the decisions to use modern family planning, as opposed to traditional methods, where they initiate about a quarter or less of the decisions. The role of wives and other people in initiating decisions relating to use of modern methods diminishes substantially (from at least 40 percent to 23 percent for wives, and from at least 33 percent to 20 percent for other people). While both men's and women's responses indicate that husbands initiate more decisions regarding use of modern contraceptives than wives and other people, a substantially higher proportion of men (71 percent) than women (48 percent) indicated that decisions to use these methods were initiated by men. These results largely show that men's control vis-à-vis their wives and other people is greater for modern methods than traditional methods. Notwithstanding the small number of cases, these patterns persist across the three culturally divergent regions. It is particularly noteworthy that husbands in the patriarchal Rumphi play a notably smaller role in initiating decisions about using traditional methods than wives and other people.

Decisions Relating to Use of Traditional Methods of Child Spacing

The qualitative data show that issues relating to childbearing are a concern not only of the conjugal couple, but of the rest of the extended family. When young couples get married, the elderly people, mostly women, monitor them closely to ensure that they start bearing children as soon as possible. Once the couple start bearing children, the next major concern for the extended family becomes whether the subsequent births are adequately spaced, and also whether the couples are adhering to various customs and rituals that are meant to safeguard the health and survivability of the young child (Zulu, 2001). When a couple have the first child, elderly women, sometimes in the company of men, come to instruct the new parents on the need for them to avoid another pregnancy while the newly born child is still very young. If the couple live in the husband's village (like in Rumphi District), it is the husband's aunt (wife to

Table 6.2
Percentage of Ever-Married Contraceptive Users by Primary Person Who Initiated the Decision to Use Contraception: TMCSM Rural Areas

PERSON INITIATING DECISION TO USE CONTRACEPTION	AREA AND SEX OF RESPONDENT											
	RUMPHI			MCHINJI			CHIRADZULU			ALL AREAS		
	Female	Male	All	Female	Male	All	Female	Male	All	Female	Male	All
EVER USE OF TRADITIONAL CONTRACEPTIVE STRINGS												
Wife	69.2	36.8	50.0	43.8	30.2	37.6	31.2	66.7	36.8	45.2	33.3	39.9
Husband	15.4	0.0	6.2	20.3	35.8	27.4	43.8	0.0	36.8	23.7	25.3	24.4
Other	15.4	63.2	43.8	35.9	34.0	35.0	25.0	33.3	26.3	31.2	41.3	35.7
Cases	13	12	32	64	53	117	16	3	19	93	75	168
EVER USE OF TRADITIONAL ORAL CONTRACEPTIVES												
Wife	63.6	30.0	47.6	54.6	30.0	38.7	75.0	–	60.0	62.2	29.3	44.9
Husband	22.7	20.0	21.4	9.1	35.0	25.8	–	–	–	16.2	26.8	21.8
Other	13.6	50.0	31.0	36.4	35.0	35.5	25.0	100.0	40.0	21.6	43.9	33.3
Cases	22	20	42	11	20	31	4	1	5	37	41	78
CURRENT USE OF MODERN CONTRACEPTIVE STRINGS												
Wife	16.7	0.0	13.3	66.7	22.2	33.3	30.0	0.0	25.0	28.0	14.3	23.1
Husband	50.0	66.7	53.3	33.3	66.7	58.3	50.0	100.0	58.3	48.0	71.4	56.4
Other	33.3	33.3	33.3	0.0	11.1	8.3	20.0	0.0	16.7	24.0	14.3	20.5
Cases	12	3	15	3	9	12	10	2	12	25	14	39

father's eldest brother) and grandmother who give young couples instructions on various issues relating to reproduction. If the couple live in the wife's village (like in Chiradzulu), however, it is the woman's aunt (mother's sister) and maternal grandmother who perform this role. Elderly men do not normally get involved in reproductive matters; their main concern is to ensure that the man works hard, and is capable of making all necessary provisions for the family such as food, housing, and other essentials. In Rumphi the couples are instructed to abstain until after the woman resumes menstruation, while in Chiradzulu they are advised to abstain for about 6 months, and in Mchinji for about 3 to 6 months. The average durations of abstinence were 15, 9, and 6 months in Rumphi, Chiradzulu, and Mchinji, respectively (Zulu, 2001).

Although it is generally argued that observing postpartum abstinence is important for the child's health, many people in the three communities acknowledged that it is not easy to abstain from sex for the prescribed durations. Many women complained that their husbands force them to have sex during the abstinence period, sometimes even beating them if they continue resisting. Indeed, while early resumption of intercourse is mostly caused by men's pressure, it is the woman who is ridiculed by her friends and elders when she gets pregnant too soon after giving birth. She is seen as a possessive woman who could not live with the prospect that her husband would go to other women during the abstinence period. Thus, it is actually the woman who takes the greater responsibility to ensure that births are adequately spaced. The excerpts below show the extent of men's influence in initiating early resumption of sex:

> We were told to wait for six months before meeting with my husband again, but after the birth of our second child we started having sex after three months. My husband was pestering me a lot. For me it was okay to wait because most of the time when a woman has just given birth she does not have the desire to have sex. [Thirty-two-year old woman, Mlonyeni, Mchinji]

> My husband was not understanding and he did not like to abstain from sexual intercourse. As a result he beat me up all the time I refused him to have sex with me. I reported to the elders but all they advised me was to persevere. [Focus group discussion for middle-aged women, Rumphi]

Couples who seek to delay pregnancies beyond the time they resume intercourse may use traditional methods such as contraceptive strings and herbal medicines. During the qualitative study we asked people who had used the methods how they got to use the methods, and who played a key role in getting them to use the methods. The data revealed that particularly women who get pregnant too soon after resuming intercourse, or who have birth complications that warrant them to have extra rest before having another child, have traditionally used these methods for emergency purposes. As such, traditional methods are usually considered for use after the second or third birth when women have enough intervals to evaluate how long the woman takes to get pregnant after resuming intercourse and menstruation. If the woman takes a longer time to get pregnant, she is regarded as a "natural spacer," and hence, not considered a candidate for birth-spacing methods when the couple resumes intercourse. However, if the woman gets pregnant soon after resuming sex, she is described as one with "soft tubes." The following excerpts from the qualitative interviews show how people get to decide to use the methods:

Yes, we are taught about traditional methods. When the first child is born parents don't necessarily talk about family planning. However, when they note that you become pregnant again while the child is still very small, that's when they fetch you medicine for child spacing. There are different types of medicine. Some tie a string around the waist. [Focus group discussion for young women, Mchinji]

It's because of the way I was created; I get pregnant within a short period. I learnt about traditional medicines from an elderly woman in the village. They were asking me why I was having children so close to each other. They then advised me to go to a herbalist so that I can get medicine for spacing. If a woman gives birth after one year like myself, she can get medicines so that she can rest for another year before getting pregnant again. [Twenty-two-year-old woman, Chiradzulu]

Although men sometimes get involved in making decisions regarding use of traditional methods, it is the elderly women who play a leading role in recommending or providing the methods to women. In some cases, the elderly women can even provide a contraceptive method to a woman without necessarily asking her or her husband whether they would like to use the method. The following excerpt demonstrates the dominant role that elderly people, especially women, play in determining use of these methods:

It was a very painful experience for me. When I later came here [from the town where husband works] I was still very weak. My grandparents took me to the hospital. But before they took me to the hospital, they tied a string around my waist. I asked them what the string was and what it meant. They told me it was to prevent me from getting pregnant soon. That's how I knew the medicine. [Focus group discussion for middle-aged women, Chiradzulu] .

Decisions Regarding Use of Traditional Medicines for Abortion and Sterilization

Many people, particularly elderly women, consider induced abortion reprehensible. Most elderly people are against abortion not only because of their "prolife" alignment, but also because of the understanding that women usually resort to abortion because of careless and irresponsible behavior. For instance, women are likely to resort to abortion if they have been unfaithful to their husbands, or they failed to adhere to postpartum sexual abstinence and conceived while the last child is still very young, or (for girls), they got pregnant before they got married or while in school. Induced abortion has traditionally been reserved for situations where the woman's life is endangered by the pregnancy. Several elderly women we talked with told us that as a way of punishing women for the irresponsibility, they deliberately provide wrong medicine so the abortion fails. As the following excerpt from an interview with a traditional birth attendant in Rumphi shows, a woman wanting to have an abortion may be given traditional medicine meant to guard against miscarriage or abortion so that she fails to abort.

> I have heard that when some women get pregnant when they still have a very small child they agree with their husbands to abort using traditional medicines that they drink. But in my opinion, that is bad. If such a person comes to seek medicine for abortion from me I would give him/her medicine that would prevent the abortion by any means. [Traditional birth attendant, age unknown, Rumphi]

This stance is advocated as the best way to teach the "disobedient" younger generation by letting them experience the problems associated with giving birth to a child that they are not ready to have.

Unlike other traditional methods of birth spacing, medicines that are used for abortion are generally considered to be very effective, although commonly with fatal consequences for women. Most transcripts have examples of women, particularly schoolgirls, who became sterile, got seriously sick, and died because of complications resulting from abortions. Because abortion is commonly regarded as a risky undertaking, and because couples are required to observe some period of sexual abstinence following an abortion, a married woman's decision to have an abortion has to be made in consultation with the husband.

People in our study sites have various traditional medicines that are used for stopping childbearing in cases where childbearing endangers the woman's life, or when the woman has too many children due to multiple births. Stopping childbearing before a woman attains menopause is considered an unfortunate event, and is normally perceived with suspicion in the traditional setting. The couple is suspected to have violated a taboo (like having sex during a funeral ceremony), or contracted a sexually transmitted disease. Development of secondary sterility is also commonly attributed to witchcraft. In fact, almost all the women who told us that they stopped bearing children at a relatively young age claimed that they had been bewitched. The following excerpt shows the nature of considerations that come into play when the decision to terminate childbearing is contemplated:

> Some women always have problems when delivering, others even take three days of labor before giving birth! To save such women from dying they are given some medicine to stop giving birth. [Focus group discussion for old men, Mkanda]

If the woman's circumstances dictate that she should be sterilized, elderly women would typically consult with elderly men and the husband to have the woman sterilized. Just as with abortion, sterilization cannot be effected without the knowledge and consent of the husband, and as the following excerpt shows, many men are opposed to it:

> The medicines are there but the elderly women who can give out these medicines cannot give them to women without the consent of their husbands. That is the problem. In most

cases, husbands cannot allow their wives to be closed, even when the woman's life is in danger due to childbirth. [Focus group discussion for middle-aged men, Rumphi]

Decisions Relating to Use of Modern Methods

After banning the provision of modern family planning services in all government hospitals in 1969, the Ministry of Health started providing family planning services in its establishments in 1984. Family planning services are mostly provided by the Ministry of Health, as a component of its maternal and child health program. When the family planning program was instituted, it was officially known as the Malawi child spacing program, and women who wanted to use contraceptives were required to obtain the consent of their husbands. This requirement, which represented a substantial change from the traditional practices where planning issues relating to birth spacing were left in the hands of women and the only decisions that required men's consent related to abortion and sterilization, was dropped in 1994 when it became evident that the husband-consent requirement prevented many women from using family planning services (Malawi Government 1994).

The timing of use of contraception and gender roles in relation to decision making differ between the modern and traditional reproductive regimes in several ways. First, even first-time mothers are urged to start using contraceptives after giving birth, rather than only after they prove to have "soft tubes," as is the case in the traditional regime. Second, because the information and advice given by the clinic personnel are widely respected, health personnel are an alternative source of authoritative information about the management of reproduction. After giving birth, women are advised to come back to the clinic after six weeks for an examination. They are then told they may resume intercourse and start using contraceptives (initially condoms, and later pills) if they want to do so. The health personnel's advice thus conflicts with the traditional prescriptions regarding the duration of postpartum abstinence (Zulu, 2001) by permitting women to contravene the abstinence taboo so long as they are protected from getting pregnant.

While men generally do not question the fact that traditional methods are usually introduced in their families without their consent, they were adamant that they should be part of the decision-making process with regard to modern contraceptives. Indeed, many men would not be too upset if they discover their wives wearing contraceptive strings provided by an elderly female relative without their prior knowledge or consent. However, use of modern family planning without the knowledge and consent of the husband becomes a contentious issue.

The qualitative data demonstrate a number of reasons why men seek to be consulted before their wives adopt modern contraception. First, men seek to exert greater control on use of modern methods as a way of fulfilling their traditional role as primary decision makers on development activities and projects. Modern methods are new, they have been vigorously promoted through the local media, and they are administered by the modern health service system. Thus, modern methods are as much a symbol of modernity as employment in the formal sector, higher education, primary health care projects, and party politics. Men typically take the lead in these areas, and perhaps they feel they should also lead in the domain of modern contraceptives, as the following except from a male FGD in Rumphi demonstrates:

Some men allow their wives, while others do not, it depends on the husbands. Yes, it is important. You know, some men do not trust their women, or they do not want to appear like they are taking orders from their women. When an issue is brought into the house by the woman, it does not carry as much weight as it would if it is brought up by the man. Sometimes you may start getting suspicious about what she really wants—she may just want to refrain from sleeping with you often, those types of things. [Focus group discussion for young women, Rumphi]

Men's opposition to modern contraception may also be a manifestation of their exclusion from activities of the family planning program. Indeed, although men demand to participate in the decision-making process relating to modern contraception, they acknowledge that they do not know as much about modern methods as their wives do because of the program's exclusive focus on women, as the following excerpt shows:

I think my wife would want to use family planning because I think that she should already know the importance of having fewer children. She goes to clinics where they are taught such things. As such she may appreciate this even better than I do. In my case, I only know these things from the radio. [Twenty-two-year-old man, Rumphi]

However, considering that the traditional reproductive regime has customarily sidelined men, except in situations where decisions regarding abortion and sterilization are contemplated, it is intriguing that men consider their exclusion from the modern family planning program an issue. This suggests that there is something unique about modern methods that attracts men to crave for direct involvement and leadership. The potency of modern methods, relative to traditional ones, may be considered a key factor to men who would like to have more children than their wives. Indeed, although modern contraceptives are generally disliked because of their potential health side effects, those who opt to use them do so because of their superior effectiveness (Zulu 1998). Thus, modern contraceptives are widely considered as limiting methods, even though most of the methods promoted by the program are meant to fulfill birth-spacing needs. Considering that birth spacing has been the primary objective of the traditional reproductive regime, one would expect greater men's approval and support to use modern contraceptives for spacing purposes. The following excerpts from FGDs in Chiradzulu demonstrate the general perception that using modern contraception is synonymous to limiting family size:

Some of us do not go to the clinic. You know what these husbands say, that if you go there you will find me gone with my blanket. So I say, why should I risk my marriage because of going to the family planning clinic? I will just go on having children; whether we have problems feeding or clothing them it does not matter. Yes, you have to continue childbearing, what else can you do? You can only go against his will if the situation is really bad, like you already have many children and you are having problems with them, but he cannot understand. [Focus group discussion for young women, Chiradzulu]

Another feature of modern contraception that seems to attract the involvement of men is the perceived link between their effectiveness of contraception and infidelity. It has been suggested that African men's opposition to modern contraception is partly driven by their fear that their wives would have extramarital affairs since there would be less risk of a telltale pregnancy (Caldwell and Caldwell 1988). Similar statements were frequently made in our focus groups and interviews, as demonstrated by the following except from a female FGD in Rumphi:

I would use modern family planning if my husband allows me to. The problem would be if my husband does not want me to use family planning. Then I would not do it against my husband's will. My husband does not want me to use contraceptives. He says those things promote promiscuity. He thinks that if he goes away for some time, I will be having sex with other men using contraceptives since there is no way he is going to know when he comes back since with contraceptive I cannot be pregnant. That's what my husband says. My husband does not want me to use contraceptives; he also says contraceptives promote promiscuity. [Focus group discussion for middle-aged women, Rumphi]

It appears strange that African men are prepared to let their wives use traditional methods without the concern that the women would be unfaithful to them. However, this makes sense given that modern contraceptives are perceived to be more potent than traditional methods (Zulu 1998), a characteristic that is bound to heighten men's anxieties that their wives would cheat on them.

Finally, the relocation of family planning services from the village to the clinic and the involvement of nurses in managing reproductive issues undermine the balance of power between the family and the outside world, and between men and women. In the traditional system, the man is assured that the elderly women would make decisions in his interests and that of the family. This is not the case with modern contraceptives, which are administered in a bureaucratic setting by uniformed nurses who cannot be presumed to be motivated by the interests of the man or his family—especially given the program's ideological shift from child spacing to a family planning program. Clinics generally proclaim that the conjugal couple should make reproductive decisions together, thus sidelining the elderly women. Modern family planning, which gives nurses a central position in managing reproductive issues, thus undermines elderly women's influence and control of their "children's" reproductive lives. During the qualitative research we learned that nurses often collaborate with women by facilitating secret use of contraception in cases where the husband disapproves (see also Rutenberg and Watkins 1997). Thus, not only do clinics undermine the role of elderly women on reproduction, their actions also contradict the program's proclamations that reproductive decisions should be made by the conjugal couple. The diminishing importance of elderly women's role on reproductive issues that is brought about by modern family planning may be part of the explanation for some of the elderly women's active opposition to modern contraception, as the following excerpt from an interview with a nurse in Rumphi shows:

> Many mothers-in-law are definitely against family planning. Some even say it here when they come with their daughters-in-law; they tell the women not to listen to our advice about family planning. What happens is that when a woman comes to deliver or to attend antenatal clinics we give them advice about what they should do after delivering. When we advise them to use contraceptives, some mothers and mothers-in-law take the women aside to tell the women to disregard what we are telling them. [Nurse, Mhuju Rural Hospital, Rumphi]

Although most women think that it is important for the husband to approve their use of modern contraceptives, there was a general understanding that the wife may have to use modern contraceptives without the husband's consent if he is lazy, and does not help her in taking care of the children. Similarly, a woman who experiences birth complications may also be justified to use modern contraceptives without the husband's consent if he does not appreciate her plight. Thus, there is a strong sense that a woman should have valid grounds before deciding to use contraceptives secretly, and that the grounds should be of the nature that even the woman's and man's parents would understand, in case her decision to use contraceptives secretly would lead to marital conflicts.

DISCUSSION

The study set out to examine the relative roles of husbands, wives, and other people (particularly the elderly) in making decisions regarding use of modern and traditional methods of family planning in Malawi, and offer explanations for differences, if any. The quantitative results show that husbands play a greater role than their wives and other people in initiating decisions to use modern methods of contraception. However, wives and other people play a greater role than husbands in initiating use of traditional methods. These results are strongly collaborated by qualitative data, which show that reproduction in the traditional context is predominantly women's domain. Elderly women (grandmothers, mothers-in-law, and aunts) make most reproductive decisions, with limited consultation with men, except when more serious decisions relating to sterilization and abortion are contemplated. When a couple gets married, the elderly women monitor them to ensure that they have a child as soon as possible. If the woman does not get pregnant soon, the elderly women suggest or prescribe treatment for the couple to undergo in order to start having children. The elderly women teach couples about the normative durations of postpartum sexual abstinence and rituals that the couple should perform before they resume intercourse. Users of traditional methods of birth spacing are usually determined after one or two births when a determination is made of how long the woman takes to get pregnant again after resuming intercourse. Traditional contraceptives may also be used when the woman has health problems emanating from birth-related complications as a way of giving her some time to rest before conceiving again.

It is important to note that the elderly women control the reproductive arena in a similar way in the matrilineal and patrilineal societies examined in this study. The difference is that it is the man's female kin who play a key role in the patrilineal communities, while it is the woman's kin who play the key role in the matrilineal (matrilocal) communities. For the most part, the husband and elderly men play a limited role on decisions relating to initiation of childbearing, the overall number of children to have, and whether to use traditional methods of birth spacing or not. The fact that decisions with antinatalist repercussions (sterilization and abortion) cannot be made without the knowledge and consent of the husband and other elderly men underscores men's dominance in reproductive decision making in these settings.

Although the administration of modern contraceptives through the maternal and child health programs ensures that modern family planning remains in the domain of women, the delivery process and decision-making dynamics change remarkably. The base for the delivery of family planning methods is relocated from the village to the clinic, where elderly women are replaced by family planning workers as instructors of potential contraceptive users, as providers of the methods, and, more generally, as the source of authoritative information regarding reproductive matters. Furthermore, men, who are content to keep a low profile in the traditional reproductive regime, are demanding to play a leading role in making decisions regarding use of modern methods.

Men's demands to have direct involvement in making decisions about use of modern contraceptives seem to be motivated by several differences in the perceived characteristics of traditional and modern methods. One is the setting in which they are provided: modern methods are provided in a modern institutional setting, and are thus associated with modernity and progress. Men are expected to play a leading role in the domain of the modern. Clinics are modern, but the integration of family planning with maternal and child health clinics makes the clinics women's spaces. Traditional methods are also administered by women, and in women's spaces, but elderly women whom the men trust administer them in the village. Second is the perceived greater effectiveness of modern contraception. Men who are suspicious about their wives may exert more control over the more effective modern methods because the women may easily get away with cheating on them. Additionally, despite the fact that most modern contraceptives are geared toward child spacing rather than family limitation, modern methods are widely regarded as birth-limiting methods. As a result, the interests of men who desire more children than their wives are threatened by the reality that use of modern family planning would allow their wives to have a more firm control on their reproductivity. This result demonstrates the need for social marketing agents to emphasize that modern contraceptives are meant to meet the needs of both spacers and limiters.

The influence of elderly women in reproduction depreciates by the relocation of contraception from the village to the clinic. However, the fact that some of the elderly women retain substantial influence regarding use of modern contraceptives suggests the need for the family planning program to pay some attention to them, and possibly exploit their influence to promote modern methods. For the most part, the elderly women are favorable to ensuring that births are adequately spaced, and involving them in the activities of the program may ease some of their opposition to modern methods. Since men are usually responsible for early resumption of sex after birth, one would expect them to be more supportive of modern family planning because the protection against pregnancy would facilitate early resumption of sex without exposing themselves to the public ridicule that is heaped on couples that do not space their births adequately.

NOTE

The authors are grateful to Susan Watkins (University of Pennsylvania), Francis Dodoo (University of Maryland), and Alex Ezeh, Gloria Chepngeno, and Salome Wawire (African Population and Health Research Center) for their useful comments on earlier versions of this chapter.

REFERENCES

Bankole, Akinrinola Stephen. (1995). Desired fertility and fertility behavior among the Yoruba of Nigeria: A case study of couple preferences and subsequent fertility. *Population Studies* 49: 317–328.

Bankole, Akinrinola, and Susheela Singh. (1998). Couples' fertility and contraceptive decision-making in developing countries: Hearing the man's voice. *International Family Planning Perspectives* 24(1): 15–24.

Becker, Stan. (1996). Couples and reproductive health: A review of couple studies. *Studies in Family Planning* 27(6): 291–306.

Biddlecom Ann E., J.B. Casterline, and A.E. Perez. (1997). Spouses' views of contraception in the Philippines. *International Family Planning Perspectives* 32(3): 108–115.

Caldwell, J.C. (1977). The economic rationality of high fertility: An investigation illustrated with Nigerian survey data. *Population Studies* 31(1): 5–28.

Caldwell, J.C., and P. Caldwell. (1987). The cultural context of high fertility in sub-Saharan Africa. *Population and Development Review* 13(1): 409–437.

Casterline, John B., A. Perez, and A. Biddlecom. (1997). Factors underlying unmet need for family planning in the Philippines. *Studies in Family Planning* 28(3): 173–191.

Dodoo, F. Nii-Amoo. (1998). Men matter: Additive and interactive gendered preferences and reproductive behavior in Kenya. *Demography* 35(2): 229–242.

Drennan, M. (1998). Reproductive health: New perspectives on men's participation. *Population Reports.* Vol. Series J., Baltimore: Johns Hopkins University School of Public Health, Population Information Program.

Ezeh, Alex Chika. (1993). The influence of spouses over each other's contraceptive attitudes in Ghana. *Studies in Family Planning* 24(3): 163–174.

Malawi Government. (1997). *Demographic and Health Survey 1992.* Calverton, MD: Macro International Inc and National Statistical Office (Malawi).

———. (1994). *The Malawi National Family Planning Strategy 1994–1998.* Lilongwe: National Family Welfare Council of Malawi.

Mbacke, C. (1994). Family planning programs and fertility transition in sub-Saharan Africa. *Population and Development Review* 20(1): 188–193.

Miller, Kate, Eliya M. Zulu, and Susan Cotts Watkins. (2001). Gender and husband-wife survey responses in Malawi. *Studies in Family Planning* 32(2): 161–174.

Omondi-Odhiambo. (1997). Men's participation in family planning decisions in Kenya. *Population Studies* 51(1): 29–40.

Rosenfield A.G., W. Asavasena, and J. Mikhanorn. (1973). Person-to-person communication in Thailand. *Studies in Family Planning* 4(6): 145–150.

Roudi, Farzaneh, and Lori Ashford. (1996). *Men and Family Planning in Africa.* Washington, DC: Population Reference Bureau.

Rutenberg, Naomi, and Susan Cotts Watkins. (1997). The buzz outside the clinics: Conversations and contraception in Nyanza province, Kenya. *Studies in Family Planning* 28(4): 290–307.

Srivastava, M.L., and W. M'manga. (1991). *Traditional and Modern Methods of Child Spacing in Malawi: Knowledge, Attitude and Practice.* Zomba: University of Malawi, Demographic Unit.

Watkins, Susan Cotts. (1993). If all we knew about women was what we read in Demography, what would we know? *Demography* 30(4): 551–577.

Watkins, Susan Cotts, and Dennis Hodgson. (1998). From mercantilists to Neo-Malthusians: The international population movement and the transformation of population ideology in Kenya. *Workshop on Social Processes Underlying Fertility Change in Developing Countries: Organized by Committee on Population, National Academy of Sciences* (Washington, DC. Jan 29–Jan 30).

Westoff, Charles F., and Akinrinola Bankole. (1998). The time dynamics of unmet need: An example from Morocco. *International Family Planning Perspectives* 24(1): 12–14.

Yinger, N.V. (1998). *Unmet Need for Family Planning: Reflecting Women's Perceptions.* Washington, DC: International Center for Research on Women.

Zulu, Eliya M. (1998). What can family planning programs learn from traditional reproductive practices and beliefs? A case study from Malawi. *IUSSP Seminar on Reproductive Change in sub-Saharan Africa* (Nairobi, Nov. 2–Nov. 4).

Zulu, Eliya M. (2001). Ethnic variations in rationale and observance of postpartum sexual abstinence in Malawi. *Demography* 38(4): 467–479.

7

THE NATURE OF UNMET NEED FOR CONTRACEPTION IN NDOLA, ZAMBIA

Ann E. Biddlecom and Frederick A.D. Kaona

INTRODUCTION

"Unmet need for contraception" refers to the desire to prevent pregnancy in conjunction with a lack of any contraceptive practice. The importance of this concept rests on the assumption that it is strongly equated with a latent demand for contraception, usually assumed to be modern contraceptives. The concept has received widespread recognition for identifying, in part if not in whole, a subpopulation of women and men who are potential contraceptive users, and presumably services and programs can respond. By addressing unmet need, programs can focus on individual fertility goals instead of national demographic targets and, as an added benefit, help reduce fertility (Sinding et al. 1994).

The work of Westoff and Bankole (1995) is one of the most comprehensive accountings of the components and levels of unmet need throughout the developing world. Other studies have addressed what the impact on fertility is of "meeting" unmet need (Bongaarts 1991; Greene et al. 1997; Westoff and Bankole 1996). Still other studies have refined the measurement of unmet need to include other population groups such as men and expand the definition of unmet need to encompass health risks or ineffective contraceptive use (DeGraff and DeSilva 1996; Dixon-Mueller and Germain 1992; Ngom 1997; Perez and Palmore 1997; Westoff 1997). What still remains relatively undeveloped is examination of the specific barriers that prevent women and men, who are otherwise interested in avoiding unintended pregnancy, from using contraception.

The determinants of unmet need have particular importance in the context of sub-Saharan Africa. Fertility rates continue to remain high in most sub-Saharan African countries and the use of modern contraception is still relatively low. Levels of unmet need among married women of reproductive age in this region range from 19 to 37 percent, and the majority of unmet need is for birth spacing rather than limiting childbearing (Westoff and Bankole 1995). While the fertility effects of meeting unmet need for spacing are thought to be negligible (see Greene et al. 1997 for an attempt at estimating these effects), understanding the reasons for unmet need will most definitely have implications for family planning program content and structure as well as the nature of reproductive change in sub-Saharan Africa.

This study presents an in-depth analysis of the nature of unmet need in an urban setting in sub-Saharan Africa, and joins a small but growing number of in-depth studies on unmet need in other countries and regions of the world. Our underlying approach is twofold: first, we examine a broad range of determinants of unmet need rather than simply hypotheses about one or two main factors; and, second, we examine how attitudes and behaviors differ between couples where the wife is using contraception and couples where the wife is classified as having unmet need. The latter approach is especially important because some factors may present problems for *both* contraceptive users and nonusers (for example, both groups may view modern contraceptive methods as causing bad health side effects, thus affecting uptake of contraceptive use as well as discontinuation). Studies using these approaches, drawing on both quantitative and qualitative data sources and including men as well as women, have taken place in the Philippines, Nepal, India, Pakistan, Guatemala, Ghana, and Zambia (Biddlecom et al. 1997; Casterline et al. 1997; Mushingeh and Kurz 1998; Population Council 1997; Stash 1995; Yinger et al. 1997). These studies are oriented around country-specific constraints, both sociocultural and programmatic, rather than the more universalistic outlook adopted (though appropriately so) in technical calculations of unmet need.

Existing studies of unmet need point to two main explanations for its existence: (1) a measurement explanation and (2) substantive disincentives to using contraceptives (Bongaarts and Bruce 1995; Casterline et al. 1997; Robey et al. 1996). The first explanation underlies the numerous studies on refining measures of unmet need. Usually the goal is to classify some part of the population that has unmet need that was previously missed, or to show how levels of unmet need change depending on how the measure is constructed. More rarely is the purpose to examine whether women with unmet need are "falsely" classified as such (see Yinger et al. 1997).

The second explanation refers to a host of indicators that represent obstacles to practicing contraception. These obstacles closely correspond with many of the conceptual frameworks of reproductive decision making and contraceptive use (see Beckman 1983; Nag 1984; Shedlin and Hollerbach 1981). The primary obstacles to contraceptive use are: (1) weakly held fertility preferences; (2) lack of knowledge about contraceptives; (3) high costs of using contraception; (4) spouses' fertility preferences, knowledge, and perceived costs of contraception; and (5) the nature of spousal communication and decision making on reproductive matters.

How much of a barrier husbands are to women's contraceptive use, especially in sub-Saharan Africa, is still an open question, and men are often portrayed in a far more negative light than what existing evidence supports (Greene and Biddlecom 1997). Relatively few women, in fact, cite their husband's opposition as the *main* reason why they do not use contraceptives, despite their desire to delay or stop childbearing. In an analysis of unmet need in twenty-seven countries, Westoff and Bankole (1995) show that between 0 and 12 percent of married women said their partner's opposition was the main reason why they did not intend to use contraception (this figure was 9 percent in Zambia). However, men's roles in contraceptive decisions may depend on the method in question. Findings from an in-depth study in Malawi show that men have played a limited role in decisions to use traditional methods of contraception, but they demand a far larger and more authoritarian role in decisions to use modern methods (Zulu and Kalipeni, this volume). We expect that husbands may be obstacles to contraceptive use on a number of different fronts: their fertility preferences, views of methods, and the way that spouses communicate and make reproductive decisions. Our aim in this study is to examine the role of husbands on all of these dimensions.

Access and quality of family planning services also figure into decisions to use contraceptives. We do not examine access and quality in this study for two reasons. First, we chose a study setting where availability and access to contraception are not critical problems (a more detailed description of the service environment is provided in the next section). Second, an assessment of the role of services is better grounded if it is based on direct measurement of accessibility and quality of family planning services: our study data come entirely from population-based samples of men and women.

The three specific research questions we examine about the nature of unmet need are:

1. Do weak or conflicting fertility preferences distinguish women who use contraceptives ("met need") from those with unmet need?
2. Do the broad array of costs of contraceptive methods (such as social acceptability, health side effects, or financial costs) preclude the use of contraception even when there is the motivation to use?
3. Does the style of spousal communication and decision making about reproductive matters distinguish women who use contraceptives from those with unmet need?

The next section describes the setting of this in-depth study in urban Zambia and the different sources of data collected and analyzed. Evidence for each of the specific research questions described above then follows. The chapter concludes with programmatic implications of the findings and larger questions about the nature of unmet need for contraception in sub-Saharan Africa.

THE STUDY SETTING

This study was conducted in urban Ndola district, a major urban center in the Copperbelt province of Zambia, a country where nearly half of the population resides in urban areas. The city of Ndola developed as an industrial and commercial center and in 1932 it became the provincial capital city. As is indicative of the name Copperbelt province, there are a number of active mines throughout the area: the mining activity currently taking place in Ndola is copper smelting and open cast mining.

Ndola residents live in communities known as townships or compounds. These townships are run by the city council. In the mining areas, the mining companies have in the past provided accommodation for those they employed, and most of these employees had their families coresiding with them. In the late 1990s homes owned by mining concerns were sold to the sitting tenants. The mining industry in this area does not draw on large camps of male migrant laborers as is the case in other southern African nations. However, with the increasing rural-urban migration Zambia has been facing since independence, the municipal councils have not been able to cope with the provision of housing. This has resulted in the creation of unauthorized settlements known as shanty compounds or squatters. Our study design explicitly covered 14 of the 21 compounds that constitute urban Ndola district: 2 were shanty compounds, 2 were a mix of shanty and low class, 6 were low class, and 4 were middle class.

Fertility has been declining over the past two decades in Zambia but still remains relatively high at 6.1 births per woman (Central Statistical Office et al. 1997). Awareness of contraceptive methods (measured by the general indicator of having heard of a method) is nearly universal, even for modern methods. More than half of all married women have ever used a contraceptive method, two-thirds of whom have used a modern method. Contraceptive use has also risen in recent years from 15 percent in 1992 to 26 percent in 1996, and more than half of current use consists of modern methods (Central Statistical Office et al. 1997).

Despite these gains, there remain substantial discrepancies between women's reproductive desires and contraceptive behavior. Fully 27 percent of married women in Zambia in 1996 had an unmet need for contraception (Central Statistical Office et al. 1997). Most of this was for delaying pregnancy rather than limiting childbearing altogether. Yet there is still evidence of a frustrated desire for limiting: the wanted fertility rate in Zambia is nearly one birth below the total fertility rate (5.2 versus 6.1).

The study setting is also part of the "AIDS belt," where the AIDS epidemic is at an advanced stage (Cohen and Trussell 1996). Hence, it is difficult to consider unmet need for family planning without also considering issues related to HIV/AIDS. Zambia has an exceptionally high prevalence of HIV: 24.7 percent of pregnant women in urban areas in Zambia are estimated to be HIV-positive, according to point prevalence estimates from 1993 seroprevalence data (Stanecki and Way 1997).

Despite high levels of HIV/AIDS awareness and experience of sexually transmitted diseases (STDs) in general, preventive behaviors such as condom use are still rather low. Only 39 percent of married men have ever used a condom and 19 percent of married women in Zambia have ever had partners use a condom (Central Statistical Office et al. 1997). Condom use is viewed with mixed feelings: while condoms are recognized as preventing the transmission of disease, they are also associated with promiscuity (Rutenberg et al. 1997; Tweedie and Lemba 1996). Questions about unmet need for avoiding pregnancy as well as avoiding sexually transmitted diseases, then, are of key concern.

Though sexually transmitted diseases are not the main focus of this particular analysis, we will revisit this issue when discussing the implications of our findings.

Finally, the structure of Zambia's family planning and health services deserves mention because it has recently become decentralized, making in-depth studies such as this one more relevant for planning purposes. Health reforms were initiated in 1992 that decentralized service delivery, planning, and decision-making authority to the country's sixty-one health districts (Ministry of Health 1997). One of the three core elements of the national reproductive health plan launched in June 1997 is to meet the needs of individuals and couples for safe, effective, and affordable methods of fertility regulation of their choice. The Ministry recommended that family planning information and services be offered free by the government, that men and women of reproductive age be eligible to use family planning methods without the consent of their spouses or parents, and that the involvement of men in family planning and in responsible sexuality should be addressed through a variety of means, including counselling of men by the service provider. A broad range of methods are included in the Zambia family planning program. Data from a 1997 situation analysis study of health facilities throughout Zambia showed that the most common methods provided were the combined pill and male condoms (over 90 percent of facilities), the progestin-only pill (69 percent), lactational amenorrhea (LAM) (63 percent), natural family planning methods (NFP) (53 percent), and injectibles (50 percent) (Central Statistical Office 1997).

A variety of family planning services were available throughout the study setting of urban Ndola district. Of the fourteen compounds covered in this study, all but two had a government clinic within the compound boundaries. Residents in the two compounds that did not have government clinics had access to and utilized clinic services in nearby compounds (as reported by health personnel at those nearby clinics). Only one compound had an active community-based distributor. Private clinics, work-based family planning services, and pharmacies/medical shops were also present throughout the study area. At the time our study survey was fielded, eight government clinics had undergone additional provider training in family planning services and received supplies of Depo-Provera for administration, both activities implemented as part of a project by CARE.

DATA AND METHODS

The survey and qualitative data used in this study were designed and collected by the Tropical Diseases Research Centre (Ndola) in collaboration with the Policy Research Division of the Population Council (New York). Funds for data collection and analysis were made possible by awards from the Rockefeller Foundation and the United Nations Population Fund. Data were collected in urban Ndola district, Zambia, December 1996 to September 1997. The study design is comprised of three main elements:

1. Exploratory focus group discussions (December 1996)
2. Population-based survey (May to June 1997)
3. Follow-up in-depth interviews (September 1997)

The purpose of the six focus group discussions (FGDs) was to inform the content of the survey questionnaire and to obtain a sense of local terminology for family planning methods and concerns. The FGDs were held in convenient community places suggested when respondents were selected and were led by one moderator (a female nurse) and one *rapporteur* (a female assistant). All discussions were tape-recorded with the permission of the respondents, and were later transcribed, translated from Bemba into English, and transcripts were then checked against the tapes. We selectively draw on the focus group transcripts to illustrate particular explanations rather than subject the transcripts to separate analysis.

The population survey was a two-stage, self-weighting probability sample of married women and men living in Urban Ndola district. The sample consists of 1,860 married women aged 15–44 and 1,056 husbands. The response rate for eligible women was 90 percent. The response rate was lower for husbands (76 percent), due mainly to difficulties in tracking husbands for an interview (87 percent of nonresponse) rather than men's outright refusal to be interviewed. Husbands and wives were interviewed separately and not simultaneously as a rule given the difficulties in the field of arranging for interviews with husbands. Thus, there was some chance for discussion to occur between spouses following the first interview. Of the 1,056 husbands who were successfully interviewed, 1,035 (98 percent) were in monogamous marriages [note: polygyny is uncommon among men in urban areas of Zambia]. Of the 1,035 monogamous men, we were able to correctly match 901 (87 percent) to their wives' interview records. We use this sample of 901 couples for the following analyses.

Survey questionnaires were designed with the obstacles to contraception in mind from previous studies as well as the concerns raised and phrases used by participants in the FGDs. Topics include attachment to current fertility preferences, dimensions of the "costs" of contraceptive methods, reproductive health status, interaction with the formal health care system, and the nature of spousal reproductive decision making.

The third element of the study design consists of twenty-five in-depth interviews (IDIs) with married women and twenty-five IDIs with married men from the survey. As with the FGDs, all interviews were tape-recorded, transcribed, and translated from Bemba into English. We utilize the in-depth interviews in two ways. First, we check what was said in the IDIs about current fertility preferences and contraceptive use with what was reported by the same person in the structured survey interview. The comparison between the two sources of data is an attempt to examine the first explanation for unmet need: that unmet need is due to mismeasurement of fertility preferences or contraceptive use.

Second, we analyze the IDI transcripts as an independent source of data. Thematic codes were jointly constructed by the authors. Several transcripts were double-coded by each author and compared in order to ensure the same understanding of what the codes should encompass as well as consistent coding of all fifty transcripts. All coding and searches were conducted using the Windows-based qualitative software package Nud*ist. Each author independently analyzed the fifty coded transcripts and reached conclusions about how those with unmet need (as defined by the survey data) differed from those currently using contraceptives on the dimensions of interest. Interpretations were compared and reconciled with evidence from the transcripts when there were differences between the authors.

Table 7.1
Unmet Need and Contraceptive Use among Married Women in Urban Zambia (1996) and Urban Ndola District, Zambia (1997)

	Urban Zambia (1996)	Urban Ndola District (1997)
Total unmet need (%)	26.6	20.1
Spacing	16.9	15.0
Limiting	9.7	5.1
Total current contraceptive use (%)	33.3	44.6
(Total modern method use)	(23.6)	(25.6)
Pill	12.2	16.8
Injection	2.2	4.1
Other modern methods	9.2	4.7
(Total traditional method use)	(9.7)	(19.0)
Withdrawal	3.0	9.2
Rhythm/abstinence	3.0	4.9
Other traditional methods	3.7	4.9
N	1,972	901

Sources: Zambia Demographic and Health Survey, 1996 and TDRC Unmet Need Survey, 1997.

EVIDENCE

Levels of unmet need and current contraceptive use status for married women are shown in Table 7.1 for our study setting and, for the sake of comparison, for urban areas of Zambia. We draw on the algorithm used by Westoff and Bankole (1995) to identify unmet need status. The components are: (1) current contraceptive use; (2) fecundity (a variable based on behavioral measures, perceived ability to physically conceive, and responses of "unable to conceive" to questions about nonuse of contraception and desire for another birth); (3) the wantedness of the last birth or current pregnancy for women who are amenorrheic or pregnant; (4) contraceptive use prior to the last pregnancy; and (5) the desire for (and desired timing of) another birth for women who are not pregnant or amenorrheic. One-fifth of married women in Ndola have an unmet need for contraception, and most of this is for spacing (15 percent) rather than for limiting childbearing (5 percent). Our estimate is slightly lower than the 27 percent for urban Zambia in 1996, and is lower for both the spacing and limiting categories. These lower figures are partly due to higher reports of current contraceptive use in urban Ndola.

Table 7.1 shows that almost twice as many married women reported using natural or traditional methods in the Ndola study compared to women in all urban areas of Zambia in 1996. Reporting differences are most pronounced for withdrawal. Similar percentages of married women reported using modern methods, though there are differences by specific method.

One argument is that unmet need is due to mismeasurement in surveys of contraceptive behavior and fertility preferences (usually captured by one or two items). We can make two points regarding the measurement explanation. First, reports of using natural or traditional methods are likely to be underestimated in surveys that draw on the standard contraceptive knowledge grid used in the Demographic and Health Surveys. After asking the respondent to name any ways or methods that couples can use to delay or avoid pregnancy, the interviewer then works down a grid asking the respondent about each method not mentioned spontaneously. The grid begins with modern methods such as the pill and injections and ends with natural methods such as withdrawal and rhythm.

In the survey in Ndola, we retained this type of grid but switched the order of method types, such that the respondent was first asked about natural and traditional methods and then about modern methods. We did this in order to reinforce the impression that the interview concerned views of and experience with *all* types of methods and not just clinic-based modern methods. Unfortunately, the aim of our study was not to test the effect of this change in measurement and we did not implement a standard knowledge grid (with modern methods listed first) among a comparable group of respondents. The results are only suggestive in that those women (and their husbands) identified in most studies as having unmet need may in fact be using natural or traditional methods. This may be especially the case in many sub-Saharan African countries where modern method use is not very prevalent and where traditional methods often play significant roles in birth spacing.

Two experiments of method ordering, similar to that described above in the Ndola study, have been conducted outside Africa in Peru and the Dominican Republic (Goldman et al. 1989; Westoff et al. 1990). Slightly more women in the Dominican Republic reported ever using withdrawal as a contraceptive method when they were interviewed using the questionnaire that listed less effective methods (including withdrawal) first. This provides some support for what we found in Ndola. However, there were no differences by method ordering in reports of ever use of methods in the Peru study.

Our second point echoes this likely underreporting of contraceptive use. We compared responses on fertility preferences and contraceptive use from the survey with those made by the same respondents in the unstructured interview transcripts. We conclude that: (1) fertility preferences are consistently expressed in both the survey and the in-depth interviews and (2) contraceptive use may still be underreported in the survey. For example, two of the six women identified in the survey as having unmet need said they were using condoms and withdrawal in the unstructured interviews, albeit the methods were sporadically used. This comparison of respondent answers between two data types is by no means a comprehensive test of measurement, but it does suggest that unmet need may be due in part to mismeasurement of contraceptive use in surveys and that current contraceptive use, especially methods like withdrawal and condom, is not necessarily captured by a yes/no question.

We now turn to the more substantive explanations for unmet need. Our discussion of the obstacles to contraceptive use will draw attention to differences between contraceptive users and women with unmet need. We do not divide the unmet need group by spacing versus limiting desires because the number of women who wish to stop childbearing altogether is quite small. However, this is a useful analytical split in general for other studies and settings. We do divide the unmet-need group by whether or not women used a modern method in the past. Given the relatively significant number of women with prior experience with modern methods, we reasoned that discontinuation is a notable phenomenon and that women with prior experience may face different barriers to use than women who have never tried using a modern method. All percentages shown for users and those with unmet need are adjusted for women's age and level of schooling. Data are from the matched husband-wife sample from the 1997 TDRC Unmet Need survey.

WEAK OR CONFLICTING FERTILITY PREFERENCES

One potential reason for unmet need is that women's and men's desires to prevent pregnancy are weak or conflicting. We present figures in Table 7.2 for two items that indicate attachment to preferences: (1) reaction if a pregnancy were to occur in the next few months (or, if pregnant, reaction upon learning of the pregnancy) and (2) if there are any circumstances under which the respondent might change his or her mind. For both items there are very small differences between users and those with unmet need. The majority of women and men across all groups would be worried about conceiving soon (or are worried about the fact of their current pregnancy) and say that they would not change their minds about their current fertility preferences.

The only significant difference by unmet-need status is among husbands of women with unmet need, many of whom would be pleased about a pregnancy in the near future. Of course, some of these men do not want to prevent pregnancy at all and want another child soon. However, the figures in Table 7.3 on conflicting fertility preferences among couples provide little support for this argument. Roughly three-quarters of husbands and wives share the same desire (and timing) for another birth, and there is no statistically significant difference in husbands' pronatalism by unmet-need status. We can conclude that husbands of

Table 7.2
Percentage of Contraceptive Users and Those with Unmet Need by Attachment to Fertility Preferences, Ndola, Zambia (1997)

	Contraceptive User	Unmet Need	
		Ever User[a]	Never User
Wife: If pregnant soon (or at time of current pregnancy) would feel:			
Pleased	6	7	8
Worried	73	65	70
Resigned/does not matter	21	27	22
Husband: If wife pregnant soon (or at time of current pregnancy) would feel: (*)			
Pleased	13	25	31
Worried	61	49	59
Resigned/does not matter	26	27	10
Wife: Would not change mind about preferences	71	73	68
Husband: Would not change mind about preferences	76	73	84
N	402	93	88

Source: TDRC Unmet Need Survey, 1997.
Note: Percentages are adjusted for women's age and level of schooling. The sample is all monogamous couples.
* $p < .01$ (chi-square statistic for differences by unmet need status).
[a] Unmet need is is further classified by whether or not women ever used a modern contraceptive method. This classification continues throughout the following tables.

Table 7.3
Percentage of Contraceptive Users and Those with Unmet Need by Spousal Differences in Desires for Another Child, Ndola, Zambia (1997)

	Contraceptive user	Unmet need	
		Ever user	Never user
Husband is more pronatalist than wife	15	20	13
Husband and wife have same desire for another child	78	72	84
Wife is more pronatalist than husband	7	8	3
N	402	93	88

Source: TDRC Unmet Need Survey. 1997.
Note: Percentages are adjusted for women's age and level of schooling. The sample is all monogamous couples.

women with unmet need are less resistant to risking an unintended pregnancy than husbands of women who use contraceptives.

Our analysis of the in-depth interview transcripts also provides some support for the argument that women with unmet need and their husbands differ from contraceptive users in the relative strength of their fertility preferences. While both groups were explicit about their current desires to avoid an unintended pregnancy, those with unmet need expressed more fatalism about their situation. These points are exemplified by the following interview with a thirty-two-year-old woman with four children who was classified as having unmet need (limiting):

> Interviewer: Now what are you doing about it since it is not alright about children, preparing for their school and seeing that they learn properly? What are you doing about it?
>
> Respondent: Nothing [laugh]. We are waiting that we should stop having more children. God willing maybe we can look after them instead of just bearing more.
>
> Interviewer: Okay, so how many children would you like to have altogether?
>
> Respondent: No, just these are enough.

Women with unmet need and their husbands also had vaguer long-range plans for childbearing (i.e., not certain about the total number of children they wanted) and were less specific about the bad effects of the economy that they felt.

COSTS OF CONTRACEPTION

Does the broad array of costs of contraceptive methods preclude the use of contraception even when there is the desire to prevent pregnancy? We asked a number of questions about the social acceptability and health problems associated with contraceptive use in general. We also employed a matrix of questions covering a range of costs for five of the most commonly known modern and traditional methods in Ndola [pill, injection, condom, traditional string (*impimpi*), and withdrawal]. We coded responses similarly—highlighting negative perceptions of contraceptive methods—in order to make comparisons more clear.

Figures for men's and women's views of the costs of contraceptive methods are shown in Table 7.4. Few men and women disapprove of contraceptive use in general, and there are no distinctions by unmet need. Perceptions of relatives' approval do seem to play a role in unmet need: women with unmet need and their husbands either have more negative views of what relatives think about contraception or they simply do not know the views of their relatives.

Health side effects are often mentioned in the literature as a common reason for nonuse of contraceptives (Nag 1984; Robey et al. 1996). Health side effects may influence use through actual experience of side effects from previous episodes of use, anxiety about expected side effects due to rumors or hearsay, or knowledge that side effects of available or common methods are known to be contraindicated for certain women (e.g., high-dose oral contraceptives for women with high blood pressure). All questions were asked of women and men regardless of their current contraceptive use status.

The patterns in Table 7.4 suggest that perceptions of health side effects play a limited role in unmet need. The differences are negligible for whether the respondent thinks one or more methods have bad health side effects or for whether the respondent knows of friends or family who have experienced health side effects. At the same time, we must note that perceptions and hearsay of health side effects are relatively high for *all* groups of women and men. Finally, one-third or more of past *and* current contraceptive users said they had experienced some health side effects.

There are also differences by unmet-need status for other costs of contraceptives but in the *opposite* direction than what we would expect of obstacles to contraception. More users than women with unmet need reported that one or more contraceptive methods affected the enjoyment of sex, were ineffective, or were expensive to obtain. This raises the issue of the endogeneity of consciousness of contraceptive costs. Those who use contraceptives may be more mindful of the financial costs or the effectiveness than those who are not using contraception. Or perhaps use-oriented costs of contraceptive methods (e.g., financial cost) are more salient for those who are using (or have ever used) than are costs that are more social in nature (e.g., acceptability).

Table 7.4
Percentage of Contraceptive Users and Those with Unmet Need by Spousal Views of Costs of Contraceptives, Ndola, Zambia (1997)

	Contraceptive User	Unmet Need	
		Ever Use	Never Use
Social acceptability			
Wife disapproves of contraception in general	3	3	7
Husband disapproves of contraception in general	6	8	11
Wife perceives relatives disapprove (**)	12	17	13
Wife does not know relatives' views	18	16	34
Husband perceives relatives disapprove (*)	7	11	17
Husband does not know relatives' views	32	28	31
Health side effects of methods			
Wife: 1+ methods have bad side effects	89	92	87
Husband: 1+ methods have bad side effects	81	82	71

Continued

	Contraceptive User	Unmet Need	
		Ever Use	Never Use
Wife knows people who experienced bad effects	64	68	74
Husband knows people who experienced bad effects	51	49	45
Wife experienced bad effects (**)	37	46	3
Husband knows wife experienced bad effects (**)	31	35	7
Other costs			
Wife: 1+ methods affect enjoyment of sex (**)	59	54	29
Husband: 1+ methods affect enjoyment of sex	63	69	52
Wife: 1+ methods are expensive to obtain (**)	46	32	28
Husband: 1+ methods are expensive to obtain	29	37	26
Wife: 1+ methods are ineffective	37	34	27
Husband: 1+ methods are ineffective	36	39	26
N	402	93	88

Source: TDRC Unmet Need Survey, 1997.
Note: Percentages are adjusted for women's age and level of schooling. The sample is all monogamous couples.
* .01 < p < .05 ** p < .01 (chi-square statistic for differences by unmet need status).

Results from our separate analysis of the in-depth interviews suggest that women with unmet need and their husbands were much less expressive about the costs of contraceptive methods, both modern and traditional, than were users. The exception remains the health side effects of methods, especially the oral contraceptive pill.

> *In-depth interview with a thirty-three-year-old woman with five children, using injection:*
> Respondent: Anyway there was another friend of mine who usually had abdominal pain each time she took the pill until the husband stopped her. As for me I have never had problems and they truly work.
>
> Interviewer: Do you intend to keep on using family planning even in future?

> Respondent: On my own I would like to continue but I hear if you continue with the injection for over five years, it can destroy your uterus. But my worry is what I should do.

Health side effects appear to be the most important concern characterizing those with unmet need (especially those who have tried modern methods in the past) as well as those who currently use. Yet health effects of methods do not distinguish those with unmet need from those who use. All other costs do not seem to be formidable barriers to use either.

SPOUSAL COMMUNICATION AND DECISION MAKING

Table 7.5 presents figures for a number of indicators of spousal communication and decision making. Lack of spousal communication about the number of children to have or family planning methods primarily characterizes women with unmet need. However, these relationships are plagued by problems of causality and hence we hesitate to draw any firm conclusions based on these two indicators of spousal communication. For example, it is not clear whether a husband and wife first talked about using contraception and then the wife began using the pill or whether the wife began using the pill and this prompted the couple to talk about contraceptive use. Other aspects of communication and decision making measured in the survey show no statistically significant differences between users and women with unmet need. Women with unmet need are slightly more likely to perceive their husbands as being difficult to approach about the topic of family planning and to anger if approached. Most women say that these decisions are the joint responsibility of husband and wife.

The unstructured interview transcripts highlighted subtle rather than stark differences in spousal communication and decision making by unmet-need status. While both users and nonusers agreed that the husband should have final approval of contraceptive use and that relatives and friends do not have the right to advise, the process of decision making was quite different. Those with unmet need seemed to guess about what their spouses wanted or thought, whereas among those who use there was more open communication and the perception that they shared the same opinions with their spouses.

Table 7.5
Percentage of Contraceptive Users and Those with Unmet Need by Spousal Communication and Decision Making, Ndola, Zambia (1997)

	Contraceptive User	Unmet Need	
		Ever user	Never User
Never talked with husband about number of children to have together (*)	25	30	40
Never talked with husband about contraceptives (**)	12	15	32

Continued

	Contraceptive User	Unmet Need	
		Ever user	Never User
Difficult to approach husband about contraceptive use	9	10	13
Husband likely to anger if approached about contraceptive use	12	16	19
Wife's view of who is responsible for delaying pregancy:			
Both husband and wife	52	47	42
Wife alone	34	37	41
Husband or others	14	16	17
N	402	93	88

Source: TDRC Unmet Need Survey, 1997.
Note: Percentages are adjusted for women's age and level of schooling. The sample is all monogamous couples.
* .01 < p < .05 ** p < .01 (chi-square statistic for differences by unmet-need status).

In-depth interview with a twenty-five-year-old woman with two children; unmet need is spacing:
Interviewer: Does your husband know that you want to have the next child next year?

Respondent: Yes.

Interviewer: That means you have talked about it.

Respondent: (laugh)

Interviewer: (laugh) That is what I mean, you at least talked about it. That means you have talked about it, not so?

Respondent: It is just knowing.

However, it could be that the reason why those with unmet need are less likely to communicate with their spouses is that they perceive differences of opinion and do not want to bring about problems. In short, silence (and lack of contraceptive action) is the resulting solution.

CONCLUSION

Levels of unmet need remain high in sub-Saharan Africa despite recent rises in contraceptive use. As fertility transitions take root throughout sub-Saharan Africa, desired family size will decrease and both unwanted childbearing and unmet need will rise as a result if program efforts are not intensified (Bongaarts 1997). Even in the study setting of Ndola, where nearly half of married women reported using contraceptives, 20 percent were still identified as having an unmet need for contraception. One necessary action to improve family planning programs and services is to understand what underlies unmet need.

While numerous studies have set out to refine the measurement of unmet need, this study joins a small but growing literature examining the determinants of this common gap between attitudes and behaviors. We found that underreporting of contraceptive use plays some role in unmet need, though we could not make a firm determination of how much. Of the various substantive obstacles to contraceptive use, weak attachment to fertility preferences, lack of perceived social approval for contraception, and a lack of spousal communication about reproductive matters all play a role. Differences between users and those with unmet need were not very dramatic for any of these factors. In fact, it is surprising how *few* differences there were between the two groups compared to in-depth studies in other countries that followed similar analytical approaches (Casterline et al. 1997; Population Council 1997). However, a lack of striking differences was also echoed in another Zambian study on unmet need (Mushingeh and Kurz 1998). This suggests that changes implemented by family planning programs in settings like Ndola will affect many women and men in similar ways, regardless of contraceptive use status; in short, "a rising tide lifts all boats."

Based on our findings, we can make the following policy and program recommendations. First, family planning programs should place importance on both women's and men's concerns about the health side effects of different modern methods. Specifically, mass communication and community-based education efforts should warn women and men of the dangers of hearsay and direct them to sources of correct information about how methods work and the health side effects of methods. The Zambian government is already taking some steps in this regard with public media messages in English-language newspapers aimed at encouraging people not to listen to gossip (*kachepa*) and to discuss concerns with health providers instead. At the clinic level, concerns about health side effects of using contraception should be addressed through (1) an emphasis on increased method choice, (2) provider counseling about potential side effects to adopters, and (3) follow-up counseling to those who experience side effects. This is especially important given the widespread fears of one of the most common methods available in Zambia, the oral pill.

A second recommendation is that men need to be more informed and educated about the family planning and reproductive health concerns that both they and their wives and sex partners face. Men should be targeted as a group, separately from women, for discussion of health-related issues (sexual and reproductive) and ways of being a supportive partner. When the preliminary results from this research were presented locally in "community feedback meetings," many participants urged that family planning information be provided to men through existing Neighborhood Health Committees. The Committees provide a natural outlet situated *within* urban areas for men to gather together to learn about family planning and reproductive health. One advantage of these Committees as a vehicle for reaching men, as opposed to clinics, is that they are not bound to a fixed site. The meetings can be convened in a variety of places and times. This is especially important because of the difficulty of bringing men together due to their work hours and leisure activities. Moreover, while maternal and child health clinics are viewed as being exclusively for women, men are considered legitimate participants in Neighborhood Health Committee meetings.

Another approach to reach men is at the level of the couple. A number of efforts have been made to involve husbands and wives together in formal family planning activities with varying degrees of success (see Becker 1996 for a review). While we support this type of approach in general, it remains to be seen whether desired programmatic outcomes can be achieved in a more cost-efficient manner through community-wide initiatives to involve men, as described above, versus couple-oriented programs.

We would like to conclude this study with several related points about the nature of unmet need for contraception that have particular importance for Zambia, and perhaps wider implications for other sub-Saharan African countries. The extent of extramarital sexual relations and the high prevalence of HIV and other STDs in this country make contraceptive use for the purpose of disease prevention (for both the husband and wife) an important consideration in addition to pregnancy prevention. According to our survey data, 16 percent of husbands interviewed said they were currently in a sexual relationship with a woman other than their wife, among whom 43 percent were not using any contraceptive method in those relationships. Moreover, 42 percent of married men said they had had an STD (the majority identified it as syphilis or gonorrhea). Risky sexual behaviors of married men and associated health consequences do not occur without the awareness of their wives: fully 34 percent of the married women in the Ndola survey said they felt themselves at moderate or great risk of getting HIV/AIDS.

The outlook for increased condom use within marriage is not promising. A study based on qualitative data in the same setting found that "if the partner is not insisting, men prefer to forgo the condom to increase their pleasure or save money" (Rutenberg et al. 1997). This presents a critical situation where the level of extramarital sex is not negligible and a sizable proportion of those involved in extramarital sexual relationships are having unprotected sex in a setting where HIV levels are at extremely high levels. Our own analysis of the in-depth interview transcripts revealed that both those who use contraceptives and those with unmet need advocate "behaving well" as the only way to avoid STDs. Condoms still remain taboo for use within most married couples. Perhaps if condoms were mass-marketed not only as a way to avoid disease but as one of the most important ways a man can ensure the welfare of his children, men might be more willing to use condoms in outside sexual unions as well as within marriage. The association of condoms with promiscuity is still not avoidable though.

Another relevant point is that women with unmet need may be willing to risk an abortion rather than have to use a contraceptive method consistently. In essence, this is a postconception rather than a preconception solution to satisfying fertility preferences, and carries with it very stark health risks.

Focus group of women who use contraceptives:

There are many who are aborting, but you cannot know them. This is done in secrecy, you just see her in pains, when you ask what the problem is, she will always say nothing. [Laugh, and she continues], she cannot tell you after all, these children know most of the medicines. They are doing this after having had an experience from their friends. That is how some of them are dying.

In-depth interview with a twenty-seven-year-old man with three children:

If I say that the pregnancy should be taken out, she might die. So many things happen following an abortion. Just because the child is still too young and the neighbors will laugh at us saying look at them, they have just had a baby and she is pregnant already. Let us have an abortion. Sometimes it works well but we must not make it a habit because tomorrow things might not work well.

Zambia has one of the more liberal abortion policies in Africa, where it has been legal since 1972. Abortion is allowable in cases where the mother's physical or mental health is in danger; in the case of rape or incest; in the case of a risk of serious congenital abnormalities or disease; or if another child would represent a risk to the physical or mental health of existing children (note: Zambia is one of the few African countries where abortion is legal on the basis of the social welfare of existing children) (Turkson 1994). Of course, there are severe limitations to getting a safe abortion since obtaining the requisite signatures of *three* doctors (one of whom must be a psychiatrist) is well beyond the reach of most Zambians apart from the highly educated and wealthy. Future research should examine the degree to which abortion, particularly illegal abortions (or home-based attempts), substitutes for the use of contraception.

In sum, factors underlying unmet need in this population are quite different in nature than those facing West African and rural East African populations, where the social legitimacy of contraception is likely to be lower, the substitution of modern methods for postpartum behaviors a more prominent part of the changing reproductive regime, and the costs (broadly writ) of contraceptive methods much less a part of the decision to use contraception. For example, the median duration of postpartum abstinence in Zambia—4.7 months—is relatively short compared to most other countries in sub-Saharan Africa (Central Statistical Office et al. 1997). And while natural and traditional methods still constitute a sizable proportion of current contraceptive use, a substantial proportion of married women and men in Zambia have had prior experience with using modern methods. In sum, the nature of unmet demand for contraception and the programmatic solutions to help women and men avoid unintended pregnancy in Zambia and other countries are by no means part of a common "sub-Saharan African" pattern. However, the almost uniformly high levels of unmet need throughout sub-Saharan Africa indicate that the challenge of avoiding unintended pregnancy is most definitely a common one.

NOTE

Earlier versions of this chapter were presented at the International Union for the Scientific Study of Population seminar "Reproductive Change in sub-Saharan Africa," Nairobi, Kenya, November 1998 and the Annual Meetings of the Population Association of America, Chicago, Illinois, April 2–4, 1998. The study was supported by grants from the Rockefeller Foundation and the United Nations Population Fund. The authors gratefully acknowledge the comments of John Casterline.

REFERENCES

Becker, Stan. (1996). Couples and reproductive health: A review of couple studies. *Studies in Family Planning* 27(6): 291–306.

Beckman, L.J. (1983). Communication, power, and the influence of social networks in couple decisions on fertility. Pp. 415–443 in R.A. Bulatao and R.D. Lee (eds.). *Determinants of Fertility in Developing Countries: Fertility Regulation and Institutional Influences*, Volume 2. New York: Academic Press.

Biddlecom, Ann E., Eva Tagoe-Darko, and Kubaje Adazu. (1997). Factors underlying unmet need in Kassena-Nankana district. Paper presented at the Annual Meetings of the Population Association of America Meetings, March 27–29, Washington, DC.

Bongaarts, John. (1991). The KAP-gap and the unmet need for contraception. *Population and Development Review* 17(2): 293–313.

Bongaarts, John. (1997). Trends in unwanted childbearing in the developing world. *Studies in Family Planning* 28(4): 267–277.

Bongaarts, John and Judith Bruce. (1995). The causes of unmet need for contraception and the social content of services. *Studies in Family Planning* 26(2): 57–75.

Casterline, John B., Aurora E. Perez, and Ann E. Biddlecom. (1997). Factors underlying unmet need for family planning in the Philippines. *Studies in Family Planning*, 28(3): 173–191.

Central Statistical Office [Zambia]. (1997). *Zambia Situation Analysis Study, 1997.* Lusaka, Zambia: Central Statistical Office.

Central Statistical Office [Zambia], Ministry of Health, and Macro International Inc. (1997). *Zambia Demographic and Health Survey, 1996.* Calverton, MD: Central Statistical Office and Macro International Inc.

Cohen, Barney, and James Trussell. (eds.). (1996). *Preventing and Mitigating AIDS in Sub-Saharan Africa.* Washington, DC: National Academy Press.

DeGraff, D.S., and V. DeSilva. (1996). A new perspective on the definition and measurement of unmet need for contraception. *International Family Planning Perspectives* 22(4): 140–147.

Dixon-Mueller, Ruth, and Adrienne Germain. (1992). Stalking the elusive 'unmet need' for family planning. *Studies in Family Planning* 23(5): 330–335.

Goldman, Noreen, Lorenzo Moreno, and Charles F. Westoff. 1989. *Peru Experimental Study: An Evaluation of Fertility and Child Health Information.* Columbia, MD: Macro Inc.

Greene, Diana, Akin Bankole, and Charles Westoff. (1997). The effect of contraceptive use for spacing on the length of the birth interval. Paper presented at the Annual Meetings of the Population Association of America Meetings, March 27–29, Washington, DC.

Greene, Margaret E., and Ann E. Biddlecom. (1997). Absent and problematic men: Demographic accounts of male reproductive roles. Policy Research Division Working Paper No. 103, Population Council, New York.

Ministry of Health. (1997). *Family Planning in Reproductive Health: Policy Framework, Strategies and Guidelines*. Lusaka, Zambia: Ministry of Health

Mushingeh, Chiponde, and Kathleen Kurz. (1998). Unmet need for family planning in Lusaka and Mansa, Zambia. International Center for Research on Women project report.

Nag, Moni. (1984). Some cultural factors affecting costs of fertility regulation. *Population Bulletin* No. 17. New York: United Nations.

Ngom, Pierre. (1997). Men's unmet need for family planning: implications for African fertility transitions. *Studies in Family Planning* 28(3): 192–202.

Perez, Aurora E., and James A. Palmore. (1997). Reevaluating the unmet need for family planning in the Philippines. *Asia-Pacific Population Research* 10.

Population Council. (1997). *The Gap between Reproductive Intentions and Behaviour: A Study of Punjabi Men and Women*. Islamabad, Pakistan: Population Council.

Robey, Bryant , John Ross, and Indu Bhushan. (1996). Meeting unmet need: New strategies. *Population Reports*, Series J, No. 43. Baltimore: Johns Hopkins School of Public Health, Population Information Program.

Rutenberg, Naomi, Ann E. Biddlecom, Fred A.D. Kaona, and A. Kathleen Siachitema. (1997). Reproductive decision-making in the context of HIV/AIDS in Zambia. Paper presented at the Annual Population Association Meetings, Washington, DC.

Shedlin, Michele Goldzieher, and Paula E. Hollerbach. (1981). Modern and traditional fertility regulation in a Mexican community: The process of decision making. *Studies in Family Planning* 12(6/7): 278–296.

Sinding, Steven W., John A. Ross, and Allan G. Rosenfield. (1994). Seeking common ground: Unmet need and demographic goals. *International Family Planning Perspectives* 20: 23–27.

Stanecki, Karen A., and Peter O. Way. (1997). The demographic impacts of HIV/AIDS: Perspectives from the World Population Profile: 1996. Paper presented at the Annual Population Association Meetings, March 27–29, Washington, DC.

Stash, Sharon. (1995). Reasons for unmet need in Nepal: An attempt to pick up where fertility surveys leave off. Paper presented at the Annual Meetings of the Population Association of America, April 6–8, San Francisco, CA.

Turkson, R.B. (1994). A brief overview of the legal situation regarding abortion in sub-Saharan Africa. Paper presented at the Conference on Unsafe Abortion and Post Abortion Family Planning in Africa, March 24–28, Mauritius.

Tweedie, Ian, and Musonda Lemba. (1996). *Perceptions of Health Providers, Family Planning, and Contraceptives in Zambia: Smoke that Thunders*. Baltimore: Johns Hopkins Center for Communication Programs.

Westoff, Charles F. (1997). Unmet need revisited. Paper presented at the IUSSP conference on Methods for Evaluating Family Planning Programs, May 14–16, Costa Rica.

Westoff, Charles F., and Akinrinola Bankole. (1995). *Unmet Need: 1990–1994*. DHS Comparative Studies No. 16. Calverton, MD: Macro International.

Westoff, Charles F., and Akinrinola Bankole. (1996). The potential demographic significance of unmet need. *International Family Planning Perspectives* 22(1): 16–20.

Westoff, Charles F., Noreen Goldman, and Lorenzo Moreno. (1990). *Dominican Republic Experimental Study: An Evaluation of Fertility and Child Health Information*. Columbia, MD: Macro Inc.

Yinger, Nancy V., Linda Asturias de Barrios, Hema Viswanathan, and Andrew Mushenge. (1997). Unmet need for family planning: A comparison of community-level studies in Guatemala, India and Zambia. Paper presented at the Annual Meetings of the Population Association of America, March 27–29, Washington, DC.

8

SPACE, CONTEXT, AND HARDSHIP: SOCIALIZING CHILDREN INTO SEXUAL ACTIVITY IN KENYAN SLUMS

F. Nii-Amoo Dodoo, Melissa Sloan, and Eliya Msiyaphazi Zulu

INTRODUCTION

An urbanization boom is underway on the African continent. From roughly 30 percent today, the projection is that over half of the continent will be urban by 2025. In contrast to the experience of the West, the urbanization of Africa has occurred concomitantly with economic stagnation, meaning that urbanization is associated with considerable poverty on the continent (Zulu et al. 2000; Brockerhoff and Brennan 1998). By implication, the health consequences promise to be grave. Unfortunately, the historical numerical dominance of Africa's rural population, and the notion that urban development biases disadvantage rural areas, have led to the bulk of attention and research being placed on rural Africa. Meanwhile, the urban face of the HIV/AIDS scourge coincides with an emerging recognition that significant segments of Africa's urban populations are disadvantaged, even compared to their rural counterparts, insofar as social or health services are concerned (Brockerhoff and Brennan 1998).

An illustration of the consequences of rapid urbanization can be found in Nairobi—the capital of Kenya—a city that has grown at rates exceeding 5 percent per annum since the 1970s (Obudho 1997). As a result of this level of growth and a weak capital infrastructure, roughly 60 percent of Nairobi's 2.3 million people live in slums (MDC 1993). The poverty of these settlements is glaring, with residents typically having no access to running water, electricity, working toilets, or adequate sanitation facilities. Further complicating matters is the lack of government recognition of these slums as anything other than informal settlements. The "informal" label evidences government nonprovision of public and social services, including public health facilities and schools to these settlements.

Past research suggests that people in impoverished situations may be more susceptible than otherwise to engage in sexual behaviors detrimental even to their own health (Ulin 1992; Carael and Allen 1995; Meekers and Calves 1997; Omorodion 1999). It should not be surprising then that the inordinate poverty in large segments of Africa's cities, described by some as even worse than rural poverty (Zulu et al. 2000), should coexist with rates of HIV/AIDS infection much higher than in rural Africa. This is nowhere more evident than along the east/central/south belt of sub-Saharan Africa—in which Kenya is located—where the highest global levels of HIV infection prevail, and AIDS has become the leading cause of death among adults (Caldwell and Caldwell 1993; Elias 1991; Sher 1993). Because HIV spreads primarily through heterosexual means in sub-Saharan Africa (Ministry of Health 1992; Nzioka 1994; Oyoo 1992), and behavioral susceptibility is particularly acute for the most poor, women and children in slums have become extremely vulnerable (Zulu et al. 2000). Here, marginal employment opportunities force many women and, indeed, girls into a survival strategy of exchanging sex for money to meet basic needs (e.g., food, rent, and clothing).

Given that sexual knowledge and behaviors are culturally and socially constructed (Gagnon and Simon 1973; Ortner and Whitehead 1981; Miller and Fox 1987), it should not be surprising that the environment or context in which children live can socialize them into risky sexual behaviors. At ages where they are still learning to construct their social world, children are easily influenced by what they see and hear. Where open communication about sexual matters is sparse and intergenerational discussion is virtually taboo, children and adolescents are left to glean their sexual knowledge from the social environment. Beyond being less prepared—physically and psychologically—for sex, young adolescents are less economically endowed, and more socially dependent. This will be particularly true in settings like the slums, where poverty has contributed to the fragmentation of family structures. The physical and social context of slums has also moved sex from a private activity to a publicly observed behavior, which has the effect of socializing very young children into seeing sexual activity as "normal."

Despite their vulnerability, the literature on the behavioral nexus of disease spread is relatively silent on children and young adolescents and this has serious implications, given the built-in population momentum associated with past high fertility. Almost half of the Kenyan population is aged below nineteen years (World Population Data Sheet 2000). The low age at first sexual intercourse in slums and the high risk of HIV infection even at young ages (Zulu et al. 2000) together translate into a higher risk of infection from HIV and other reproductive health ills for the young adolescents, who have even less access to reproductive health facilities because of their age.

Beyond the access disadvantage to services, the fact that the data collection systems of the demographic and health community focus on people aged fifteen and above means that there is a lack of appropriate data, which has hindered our ability to examine the relationship between behavior and health outcomes for the younger members of communities. Fortunately, a recent study in the slums of Nairobi, Kenya permits the examination of not only how poverty and sexual behaviors are related, but also how children are implicated therein. The study, titled "Sexual Networking and Associated Reproductive and Social Health Concerns: An Exploratory Study of the Urban Informal Settlements in Nairobi, Kenya," produced qualitative data collected by the African Population and Health Research Center in four of Nairobi's slums in January 1999. We use data from this study to argue here that the confluence of three sets of factors—economic stresses, physical space considerations, and a facilitating social context—serves to effectively socialize children into considering sexual activity normal, even at very tender ages.

THE DATA

Four Nairobi slums—Kibera, Majengo, Kahawa North, and Embakasi—were selected from the list of nineteen informal settlements designated by the Kenyan Central Bureau of Statistics. These slums were purposely selected with close attention to their population sizes as well as their gender, age, and marital status distributions, each of which has implications for sexual networking. Slum selection also factored in geographic spread (because of its relationship to the possibility of contamination) and ethnicity (which is known to be a significant determinant of reproductive behavior). The study sought slums with heterogeneous ethnic populations that well represented the four major ethnic groups in Kenya.

The data were collected through focus group discussions. In each slum, discussions were held separately with males and females of four different age groups (13–17, 18–24, 25–49, and 50+). Discussions were also held with community leaders and service providers, resulting in information being gathered from ten groups in each of the four slums. This chapter focuses predominantly on the data from the 13–17-year-old discussion groups, although a few quotations from the other groups are included to underscore relevant points. These statements of the youth present their perspectives on slum life, as well as on the relationship between slum conditions and sexual behavior. Rather than make definitive statements or conclusions about causal linkages, we take response similarity across slums as indicative of a set of general causes and processes associated with these impoverished contexts. The data paint a picture consistent with the notion that younger members of the community are socialized, deliberate or otherwise, into thinking that sexual behavior is normal even for people of their age. The sexualized context that children are exposed to poses great physical consequence for them in the sense that it facilitates HIV transmission, as well as infection by other sexually transmitted diseases (STDs). In the ensuing sections, we demonstrate how economic, physical, and social contexts contribute to the sexual socialization of children.

THE ECONOMIC CONTEXT

The high population densities and rapidly deteriorating economic circumstances in Nairobi mean that there is an acute lack of jobs in the slums. Indeed, even residents who can find work typically earn very low wages. Money, therefore, becomes a key bottleneck to survival, forcing people to resort to whatever means they have at hand to acquire cash. Not surprisingly, the slums are full of people selling used clothing, selling vegetables, brewing illicit alcohol (often mixed with dangerous substances such as automobile fuel or fertilizer to make it more potent and, thus, cost-effective), and selling prostitution.

Because of the destitute living conditions that slum residents must contend with, selling sex has become very commonplace. Women often sell themselves to make money because there is typically no other viable means of meeting their subsistence needs. Much of this sex-for-money activity is among women who would usually not be considered prostitutes, but who have to resort to such activity to make immediate ends meet (e.g., having sex with landlords to pay rent, or with wholesale suppliers to offset trading debts).

Indeed, the circumstances are so poor that parents sometimes resort to sending their young children out to the streets to bring home money. With little education and nothing but their bodies to trade for money, the implications of such practices are worrying:

> Now if a girl is thirteen years old or even twelve and she is told by the parent to go and search, and she goes and meets an old man like this one and she wants money and the old man wants the young girls. The old man will give money to the girl. And that child, her body is still tender and does not have energy, and this man has energy, so when they have intercourse this man will spoil the girl. The reproductive organs will be spoilt. [Majengo service providers]

Parents are really conflicted about what their daughters sometimes have to do because of poverty:

> Now you see, if you had three such rooms, which you are renting out and charge at least 500 shillings ($7.14) for each, even our daughters would stop this prostitution because we can feed them. They do this because of hunger. This is where and why they get cheated. Do you understand? [Kibera woman, age group 25–49]

> Sometimes it is we parents to blame. If I tell my daughter that I want a certain thing and she is a student and she does not have money; where will she get what I have asked for? [Majengo community leaders]

Still, the amount of money that these women and girls make from sex is extremely low. In addition, men take advantage of this money constraint to pressure women into sex, paying them as little as they can get away with.

> For instance if a woman stays/lives alone, i.e., a single mother with children, and she wants to buy her children milk, the only solution would be to look for someone with money. She sells her body and gets the 20 shillings ($0.20) to buy milk. [Kibera girl, age group 13–17]

Often, because most men themselves have little money, women end up having multiple sex partners in order to ensure that they get sufficient money for their needs.

Mainly women have many sexual partners; some have children and maybe they do not have food. They try to go to people to ask for money and they are told there is no money, she goes on from one person to another until she gets money. [Embakasi girl, age group 13–17]

The discussion groups present reports of women moving from man to man as the money runs out.

> Moderator: They [*women*] look for money?
>
> Respondent #1: And when the money finishes he is chased!
>
> Respondent #2: If she gets another man who has money. She chases this one out.
>
> Moderator: Now I am the woman, now if I see [*a man*] has money, I approach him, and he comes we stay with him, for about how long do I stay with him?
>
> Respondents: When money is there.
>
> Moderator: Just how long?
>
> Respondent #3: Even two weeks.
>
> Respondent #2: You throw his clothes out! You tell him "kwa Mbwa ni nje!" (*the dog's place is out!*).
>
> [Kahawa north girls, age group 13–17]

Indeed, the older discussions reinforce the economic motivations and the explanations for multiple sexual partnerships:

If it is money she will be given one hundred shillings [equivalent of $1.44], if that is what the lady wants. If it is my brother here, he will just pay that especially if her sees that the lady is well dressed. He knows the girl's problem is money. This girl sells sukuma wiki [cheap vegetable] and all the sukuma wiki she sells is worth that one hundred shillings that Mr. Irungu is offering. Now if she is given one hundred shillings, already she gets convinced into sex. [Kibera community leaders]

and:

Question: What about the practice of someone having more than one sexual partner? #1: They are many. #2: Yah, that is money because the money you are given by one person is not enough. #1: Yes, it is not enough you go to this one, to this one. So that you can be given more. #2: Maybe you have children here, or there is one who pays rent, there is another one who educates the children. [Kibera service providers]

One result of the prevailing economic circumstances is that sex has become commodified, a fact that young adolescents understand very well:

> Respondent: You give her and she gives you.
>
> Moderator: You give her 20 shillings [$0.28], she also gives you twenty or?
>
> Respondent #1: She should pay back.
>
> Respondent #2: She should pay with a hundred. [Prolonged laughter]
>
> Moderator: How does she pay this hundred?
>
> Respondent: Through sex. [Majengo boys, age group 13–17]

An older resident fleshes the economic nature of transactions more, referring to supply, demand, and scarcity considerations:

> I think there is no definite figure that is paid for sex because you may come here and find that women are many and they are not married, she has rented a house, and she must pay rent, she has children, she has to feed them. You see like this one she has no definite figure. When it is dry [i.e., when times are difficult] let's say around 10th onwards to 20th, that time the charges are low. The price is hiked a bit around the end of the month. [Kibera man, aged 50+]

Essentially, the demand for money exceeds supply to the extent that the market for sex is extremely responsive to money supply. As one respondent states:

> If you have money, is a sure way of having many partners. [Embakasi boys, age group 13–17]

Inevitably, with the high prevalence of HIV/AIDS in Africa, and the relative lack of education and health resources, the sex-for-money exchanges facilitate the transmission of disease. As evidenced in the excerpts above, the economic conditions of the slums contribute substantially to unhealthy practices of the residents. The adolescents in our study display a clear understanding of the economic operations (i.e., sex for money) that take place in their societies. They also know what must be done to survive the slums, and they deem it normal to have multiple sex partners.

> Moderator: Are there people with multiple partners here in your age group?
>
> Respondents: [*all*] Yes! Many! Obviously. That is normal.

Moderator: What do you mean?

Respondent #1: We exchanged chicks [*girlfriends*].

Respondent #2: People are promiscuous.

Respondent #3: Nobody can be trusted.

Respondent #4: No one can stay in one position with one partner.

[Kahawa north boys, age group 13–17]

THE PHYSICAL CONTEXT

A further complicating factor regards the physical spaces that residents live in. Poverty manifests itself such that the houses of residents preclude privacy. Dwellings are constructed of cardboard, tarpaulin, and/or corrugated tin sheets, and often consist of a single room (sometimes internally partitioned by a curtain) that is typically in the neighborhood of six feet by nine feet in dimensions. In these dwellings, an entire family often uses the single room as bedroom, kitchen, and bathroom:

The houses are like this and you know there is no privacy. There is another paper that is put called curtain, which divides "the bedroom" and "main room." The so-called bedroom is for wife-husband and children sleep on the floor of the same room. [Embakasi man, age group 25–49]

#1: I think there is no secrecy in our houses when the parents are having sex. You see a child of about fifteen years sharing the same room and only separated by a curtain. When the parents start having sex, [the children] start wondering the kind of noise the parents are doing. So they will pretend that they are asleep when they are actually hearing everything. So next time, they will want to try the same things. [Kahawa north men, age group 18–24 years]

The major problem here is the house. If people had proper houses, some things would be private Children would not be trying to imitate what they hear. Because now even children of nine years are conceiving and giving birth. It is not strange, they do give birth at nine years of age. [Majengo man, age group 50+]

One result of the absence of privacy is that children often observe parental sexual activity. Although adults sometimes take measures to create a private situation, this is essentially futile as covertness is basically impossible in such conditions.

Moderator: What do parents do?

Respondent #1: They wait for the children to sleep, then they do their things.

> Moderator: So can one hear?
>
> Respondent #2: If you hear noise, you will just listen, you cannot wake up. You wouldn't bother. [*laughter*] If it is my age mate, I wouldn't be bothered. But parents—it is a very bad story.
>
> [Kawaha north boys, age group 13–17]
>
> Respondent #1: Maybe you have bad bedding [laughter]. When you have bad beddings, for instance a mattress, the curtain will cover it.
>
> Respondent #2: In my view, it does not help at all.
>
> [Kibera girls, age group 13–17]

Even if the children get to know that parents are having sex, they just keep it to themselves. [Embakasi boy, age group 13–17]

Often parents will take measures such as having sex when children are not home or sending children out to sleep elsewhere in order to prevent the children from seeing them have sex. However, even when such measures are taken, there is no guarantee that the children will be blind to what happens.

Maybe if I add, you find like such parents, if they have a grown-up child, they borrow for her a sleeping place, there could be another grown-up girl like her. And these other parents may not care whether they have grown-up girls or not. So there is nothing that such a practice helps, because when this girl goes there, and when the other parents are doing that, she will either hear what they are saying or come to find out what is happening. And if parents were left with a small child, and you see you cannot block a child's mind. The child is also there and is listening to what is going on. [Majengo girl, age group 13–17]

Children are exposed not only to the sexual activity of parents, but also to ongoing sexual activity among unmarried people, both young and old. Problematic, too, is the fact that in the physical context of the slums, it is very difficult to find private spaces for sex. One reason for this is the extremely high population density in the slums (2,600 people per square kilometer versus 135 people per square mile in Kenya). Discussants report sexual activity as taking place in public toilets, abandoned houses or cars, roadsides, or dark alleys, and even out in the bush or grasslands surrounding the slums.

> Moderator: What do boys do when they want to sleep with their girlfriends [youth]?
>
> Respondent #1: You just stand on the road and do it.

Respondent #2: You ask for a friend's room.

Respondent #3: We go to the toilets.

Respondent #4: Even behind the houses!

Respondent #5: In the bushes!

Respondent #1: Those who are under age go to the bush.

Moderator: What do you mean by "under age"?

Respondent #1: Under 10 years, up to 13 years.

[Kawaha north boys, age group 13–17]

Because as you know this one is at her place [*i.e., the girl*] and he is at his place [*i.e., the boy*]. And also as it concerns jobs; none of them is able to afford a lodging. You find that they do such things in the open. [Majengo girl, age group 13–17]

They do it in the toilet. They do it behind the churches. [Embakasi boys, age group 13–17]

The use of public areas for sexual activity increases the exposure of others, and particularly children, to the activity in the community. The openness of this activity allows young onlookers to see their peers engaging in sex. Thus, it appears that these adolescents are learning from what they observe. By seeing the behavior that some residents engage in to survive, adolescents are reproducing the behavior of the adults in the community and adopting it to be the norm of behavior among their own age cohort.

Now in our area, when people come together, a boy and a girl they usually go to a secluded place or bushy place where even small children could see them as they are passing. Then the next day you hear children say: "Hey yesterday, I saw so and so doing this." Now you see. That one is brought straight to our children. So when they grow up they just know that this thing is okay. [Majengo girl, age group 13–17]

Thus, for the adolescents, lack of privacy translates into public advertisement. This, coupled with the lack of privacy in the home, induces children to engage in sex at young ages.

THE SOCIAL CONTEXT

The impact of slum conditions on children is critical because the young, often, simply imitate what is prevalent in the social atmosphere of their community.

In the beginning [*or long time ago*] it [*STDs*] was there but it was not widespread. But what has increased it now is the sharing of many partners. Having many partners, and maybe those partners also have other many partners. You know most people like imitating others. [Kibera girl, age group 13–17]

Children are also aware of the prostitution in their settlements.

> Moderator: What about [*the health needs of children*] ages 13–17?
>
> Respondents: AIDS
>
> Respondent #1: Prostitution.
>
> Respondent #2: Most of these people are prostitutes
>
> [Embakasi boys, age group 13–17]
>
> Moderator: How can we prevent female pregnancy before wedlock?
>
> Respondent #1: Stop prostitution.
>
> Respondent #2: You see, perhaps she is in business, if you tell her to stop, she will ask you "where will I get food and a house from, if you provide, I will stop."
>
> Respondent #3: That is a job.
>
> Respondent #1: When she tires she will stop.
>
> Respondent #4: By the third kid they stop prostitution and start looking for casual jobs. She will also be old and won't have many clients. That is when she gets jobs.
>
> [Kahawa north boys, age group 13–17]

Even if children are protected from such behaviors within the home, prostitution is so rampant in the community that it is absolutely impossible to shield young children from observing it.

And the fact is... you see if you walk in the hidden streets here in Majengo you find a woman seated on a stool outside her door. You want to tell me that the small child does not know? There are those who sell sex. When a child sees a woman sitting outside her house and then a man goes in there, and the woman follows her and they lock the door. Maybe I can control it in my house. Maybe, like me, I have my wife and two children. My children are small. I could wait until they are asleep. You see something like that! I could use all my tricks. But from the fact that my neighbor is a sex dealer, will I have helped anything? [Majengo service providers]

Further complicating matters is the fact that parents and other adults frequently use drugs or drink alcohol prior to sex. However, this only exacerbates matters because alcohol and drugs often foster violence and disrespect in sexual encounters, and reduce the chances that partners will use protection against sexually transmitted diseases. Apparently, many men deliberately drink because, in this highly patriarchal society, they feel ashamed at not being able to fulfill their "manly" obligations as providers, because of unemployment or low wages. There was also a sense that some drink to preemptively dull their sense of embarrassment about their own children watching them during sex.

Because of drunkenness some people do not care whether children are watching them and this is what contributes to spoiling children early, when they are still very young. [Kahawa north woman, age group 18–24]

You know those are the barmaids and the husbands and wives who are alcoholics. When they are totally drunk, and cannot even tell their names, then, wherever they find each other, they will just finish their business there. [Kibera girl, age group 13–17]

A community leader characterizes the same as follows:

Plus this alcoholism it has spoilt very much. You come when you are drunk, your wife is also drunk. Now you "beat the drums in front of the children" because you are drunk. We are teaching these children bad manners because of poverty. [Kibera community leader]

The use of alcohol and drugs in this context often leads to violence.

> Moderator: In the last few days, we have heard cases of husbands beating their wives and sometimes even killing them. Have such things ever happened in this place?
>
> Respondents: [*chorus*] Yes.
>
> Moderator: What causes these fights?
>
> Respondent #1: Some are caused by alcohol because maybe the husband is drunk.
>
> Respondent #2: Maybe the wife is a strong Christian while the husband takes the drugs. When he comes home, the wife will get annoyed and so they will end up fighting.
>
> [Kibera boys, 13–17]

Factors such as harsh living conditions, violence within the social context, a cultural secrecy or taboo about sexuality, and early and long exposure to overt sexual activity may influence the outcomes of children continually observing their parents' sexual activity. Learning to engage in sex at such tender ages is likely related to the high birth rates of the youth, and also to the level of unwanted pregnancies. Teenage pregnancies impede children's ability to access the already limited advancement opportunities available in these contexts (e.g., schooling), and have as a logical consequence the reported high levels of abortion.

A child gives birth to a child. [Majengo girl, age group 13–17]
There is also the problem of giving birth and strangling and throwing away, throwing in the toilet. Now, for instance, you give birth to a live child, very healthy and then you tie the child, you strangle that child, and then put the child in a sack and then throw it where there are no people. [Majengo girl, age group 13–17]

> Respondent #1: You see, promiscuity brings about problems here at Soweto. You see, population growth has been brought about by sex outside marriage. In Soweto we have lots of children born out of wedlock. This is because of sex, especially with young girls.
>
> Moderator: How serious is this problem? Why are young girls giving birth just like that?
>
> Respondent #2: They practice prostitution—as a business. When they get pregnant they even try abortion.
>
> [Kahawa north boys, 13–17]

The prevailing social conditions make children learn that sex for money, multiple partnerships, and disposing of unwanted babies are all normative in their slum contexts. Exposure to the use of sex as a survival strategy is unavoidable in the context of extreme poverty, and the result is that children see these behaviors as normative.

DISCUSSION

This chapter has investigated the linkages between extreme poverty and the unhealthy sexual practices among adolescents in Nairobi's informal settlements. Given the rapid urbanization ongoing in Africa, understanding the determinants of these detrimental behavioral practices is imperative. We have observed how the social, physical, and economic conditions of the slums combine to normalize early sexual behavior.

The evidence from the available data is that children living in the slums of Nairobi are exposed to sexual intercourse early in life and often. They learn about sex at a time when they are not psychologically or physically mature enough to fully understand or handle the implications of sexual activity. In this culture, where sexual matters are hardly discussed, children are simply learning from what they observe. Given the particular social context in which these children live, this can be extremely detrimental for the children. Exacerbating what the children learn is the fact that there is a lack of preventive education, treatment facilities, and family planning and disease prevention recourses in the ultradeprived context. Currently, the poverty of these people and their desperate need for money appears to take precedence over their health.

Understanding the roots and context of the risky sexual behaviors documented in this study is critical for programs and governments seeking to reverse the high rates of HIV/AIDS infections, particularly among young people in sub-Saharan Africa. The qualitative data from the Nairobi study clearly show the need for research and policy to address young members of communities and, specifically, those aged below fifteen years. In impoverished conditions such as those in slums, the traditional focus of services to those aged fifteen and above suggests that this very vulnerable segment of the population may be relatively overlooked. Because of the ages at which children get inculcated, the implications (of infection and/or pregnancy) can be debilitating as they raise the likelihood of school dropout, thereby further impinging upon the already stunted life opportunities of women. At the societal level, the size of the young population (and the increasing relative size of the urban poor) portends dire consequences for Nairobi, Kenya, and sub-Saharan Africa.

NOTE

The citation of the chapter authors is simply alphabetical and is not intended to reflect the relative contribution of authors; the authors retain equal responsibility for this work. This research was made possible through funding from the Rockefeller Foundation to the African Population and Health Research Center (Grant # RF 99009#199).

REFERENCES

Brockerhoff, M., and Ellen Brennan. (1998). The poverty of cities in developing countries. *Population and Development Review* 24(1): 75–114.

Caldwell, John C., and Pat Caldwell. (1993). The nature and limits of the sub-Saharan AIDS epidemic: Evidence from geographic and other patterns. *Population and Development Review* 19: 817–848.

Carael, M., and S. Allen. (1995). Women's vulnerability to HIV/STD in sub-Saharan Africa: An increasing evidence. Pp. 201–222 in Pauline Makinwa and An-Magritt Jensen (eds.). *Women's Position and Demographic Change in sub-Saharan Africa.* Liege, Belgium: International Union for the Scientific Study of Population (IUSSP).

Dodoo, F. Nii-Amoo, and Akosua Adomako Ampofo. (1998). Aids-related condom use among married Kenyan men. *African Population Policy Research Center Working Papers No. 8.* New York: The Population Council.

Elias, C. (1991). Sexually transmitted diseases and the reproductive health of women in developing countries. *Population Council Working Papers No. 5.* New York: The Population Council.

Gagnon, John H., and William Simon. (1973). *Sexual Conduct: The Social Sources of Human Sexuality.* Chicago: Aldine.

Kendall, Carl. (1995). The construction of risk in AIDS control programs: Theoretical bases and popular responses. Pp. 249–270 in Richard G. Parker and John H. Gagnon (eds.). *Conceiving Sexuality: Approaches to Sex Research in a Postmodern World.* New York: Rutledge.

MDC (Matrix Development Consultants). (1993). *Nairobi's Informal Settlements: An Inventory.* A report prepared for USAID/REDSO/ESA (No. PN-ABH-74:L). Nairobi: USAID.

Meekers, Dominique, and Anne-Emmanuelle Calves. (1997). Main' girlfriends, girlfriends, marriage, and money: The social context of HIV risk behavior in sub-Saharan Africa. *Population Services International Working Paper No. 5.* Washington, DC: Population Services International.

Miller, Brent C., and Greer L. Fox. (1987). Theories of adolescent heterosexual behavior. *Journal of Adolescent Research* 2: 269–282.

Ministry of Health. (1992). *National AIDS Control Programme: Second Medium Term Plan. 1992/1996.* World Health Organization Global Program on AIDS.

Nzioka, Charles. (1994). AIDS policies in Kenya: A critical perspective on prevention. Pp. 159–175 in Peter Aggleton, Peter Davies, and Graham Hart (eds.). *AIDS: Foundations for the Future.* London: Taylor & Francis.

Obudho, R.A. (1997). Nairobi: National capital and regional hub. Pp. 292–334 in Carole Rakodi (ed.). *The Urban Challenge in Africa: Growth and Management of Its Large Cities.* Tokyo, Japan: United Nations University Press.

Omorodion, F.I. (1999). Sexual networking among market women in Benin City, Bendel State Nigeria. Pp. 9–18 in John C. Caldwell and James P.M. Ntozi (eds.). *The Continuing HIV/AIDS Epidemic in Africa.* Canberra: Health Transition Centre, Australian National University.

Ortner, Sherry B., and Harriet Whitehead (eds.). (1981). *Sexual Meanings: The Cultural Construction of Gender and Sexuality.* New York: Cambridge University Press.

Oyoo, O. (1992). AIDS: The killer not taken so seriously. *The Daily Nation* 9, January.

Sher, R. (1993). The role of women in the AIDS epidemic. *Medicine and Law* 12: 467–469.

2000 World Population Data Sheet of the Population Reference Bureau: Demographic Data and Estimates for the Countries and Regions of the World. (2000). Washington, DC: Population Reference Bureau.

Ulin, Pricilla R. (1992). African women and AIDS: Negotiating behavioral change. *Social Science and Medicine* 34: 63–73.

Zulu, Eliya M., Alex C. Ezeh, and F. Nii-Amoo Dodoo. (2000). Slum residence and sexual outcomes: Early findings of causal linkages in Nairobi, Kenya. *African Population and Health Research Center Working Papers No. 17.* New York: The Population Council.

9

ECONOMIC TRANSACTIONS ASSOCIATED WITH SEXUAL INTERCOURSE AMONG MALIAN ADOLESCENTS: IMPLICATIONS FOR SEXUAL HEALTH

Sarah Castle and Mamadou Kani Konate

INTRODUCTION

Much attention has recently focused on the role of formal and informal prostitution in facilitating the transmission of the AIDS virus and in increasing risk factors for sexually transmitted diseases (Carael et al. 1994, Preston-White 1996). Less attention has been paid to the economic transactions that often accompany "everyday" sexual relations in sub-Saharan Africa that are not considered to be formal or informal prostitution by those involved. This chapter looks at the economic context of sexual relations among unmarried sexually active adolescents in rural and urban Mali. It explores the motivations behind the exchanges of gifts and cash, and assesses factors associated with the direction of giving and receiving. It also addresses the links between economic factors and risks for sexual and reproductive health such as having multiple or concurrent partners.

Research elsewhere in Africa has indicated that transactions involving gifts and cash characterize a large proportion of sexual encounters among unmarried young people although the evidence suggests that the phenomenon is more widespread in east and southern Africa compared with the western area of the continent. For example, Nzyuko et al. (1997) report that, along the Trans-Africa Highway in Kenya, 78 percent of adolescent girls, who did not consider themselves sex workers, exchanged sex for gifts or cash. In Malawi, 66 percent of a sample of 500 adolescent girls reported having accepted money or gifts in exchange for sex (Helitzer-Allen and Makhambera 1993). In Cameroon, 5 percent of girls aged 12–17 years and 14 percent of boys of the same age exchanged money or gifts for sex (Meekers and Calves 1996). In general, the research to date indicates that the transactions are generally unidirectional from the male to female partner. However, we will show that giving also occurs from women to men but that the reciprocity depends on the perceived status and nature of the relationship.

The financial gains involved can contribute substantially to many different domains of adolescents' lives. Indeed, for some girls, the economic rewards override the perceived sensual or emotional gains from a sexual relationship. For example, in Botswana, focus group interviews conducted by Meekers and Ahmed (1997) found that female sexual activity is often primarily motivated by economic gain. One-third of female study participants viewed sex as having no advantages whereas the majority of boys valued intercourse for the pleasure they gained and for the status with which it endowed them. For many young women, sexual relations comprise their only or principal source of income to purchase basic necessities. In Ghana, Ankomah (1996) noted that women in premarital relationships expected the partner to contribute money for food or to help pay the rent. Others used what they were given as startup capital for small businesses. The phenomenon of "sugar daddies" has been addressed in many studies in Africa. For example, in Zimbabwe, older men have been noted to entice girls for sex with the promise of presents or money (Finger 1993). Other girls may rely on gifts from partners much older than themselves to pay school fees for clothes (Aryee 1997).

The phenomenon of gift giving reflects the nature of gender roles. These govern the direction of giving between men and women and need to be viewed within the context of local customs, which require, in many African settings, that a man gives a gift or cash in order to fulfill his role as provider and to satisfy his female partner's expectations. For the latter, tradition often dictates that she acknowledges or even "spoils" her partner by giving him presents to show him that he is appreciated. Thus, gift giving may represent not only an economic consolidation but also an emotional fulfillment of a relationship between a young man and woman.

The gender-based power relations that surround economic transactions after intercourse have repercussions for reproductive health and in particular for the transmission of HIV and STDs. In Uganda, a study indicated that between the ages of fifteen and twenty-four young women were twice as likely as young men to be infected with the AIDS virus. The author concludes that this disparity is due to the age differences between the younger women and the older partners who probably infected them (Mati 1989). As older men are likely to be economically better off, girls may see them as being able to provide more lucrative financial rewards than boys from their own age group. However, they risk exposing themselves to reproductive health risks as these older male partners have been sexually active over a longer period and thus have had a greater risk of being infected with HIV than boys from the girls' own age group who have only just started their sexual lives.

ADOLESCENT REPRODUCTIVE HEALTH IN MALI

Little is known about the extent and context of the exchange of money or gifts for sex in Mali except among formal or clandestine sex workers (Plan International 1997). Among the general population, the Demographic and Health Survey (EDS, 1995-1996) noted that during the 12 months preceding the survey, 21.8 percent of all women of reproductive age had received payment in cash or kind for sex. This increased to 25.6 percent among unmarried 15–19-year-old girls. Married women aged 15–49 reported far fewer exchanges, with only 4.9 percent admitting that they had been financially reimbursed after sexual relations. It will be discussed below that girls who are formally engaged or married tend to receive such payments less frequently than their unmarried counterparts. In such relationships, sexual relations are perceived to be part of the conjugal contract and male partners are thus not obliged to directly reimburse their spouses or fiancees for sex but rather ensure that their day-to-day material needs such as food and clothing are catered for within their marital unit.

The Demographic and Health Survey also showed that, among unmarried men of all ages, 30.6 percent reported giving cash or a gift in exchange for sex over the last year. This decreased to just 4.8 percent of married men for the reasons described above. However, the distinction between those giving to formal prostitutes and those reimbursing girlfriends or more regular partners is not clear from the data. Among sexually active unmarried men aged 15–19, the proportions giving such reimbursements fell to just 19.2 percent probably because, compared with older men, they lack the financial means to provide such rewards and are likely to have intercourse with younger partners who are less financially demanding.

Interestingly, the Demographic and Health Survey showed that the proportion of women (of all ages) receiving reimbursement for sex increased with educational level. Eighteen percent of those with no education had reported receiving reimbursement compared with 26.2 percent of those with at least a secondary education. This may be because educated women choose educated partners who have greater earning power and more resources with which to compensate them. However, the survey also indicated that increased education among men appeared to make them less likely to give a gift to their partner(s). Twenty-six percent of men with at least a secondary education had given a gift or cash over the last year compared with 32.7 percent of those with no education. Given that female school enrollment is fairly low in Mali, it may be that educated men have sexual relations with women less educated than themselves. Compared with their educated counterparts, these women may not be so demanding financially and perhaps seek other long-term benefits such as marriage rather than immediate financial rewards.

STUDY DESIGN

The survey discussed here took place in the cities of Bamako and Mopti and in the rural areas of Kolokani and Kolondieba. A total of 775 boys and 921 girls aged 15–19 were interviewed about their current and past sexual activity, reproductive health (including knowledge and use of family planning), and knowledge and experience of STDs. In addition, a locally appropriate psychological test was administered to assess their degree of self-esteem and assertiveness and to measure locus of control. Thirty focus group discussions were also carried out in rural and urban areas to elicit qualitative information about the context of adolescents' first and subsequent sexual encounters. The focus groups were translated and transcribed and analyzed using the Ethnograph computer software.

CHARACTERISTICS OF SAMPLE

All but 15 boys were unmarried, while among the girls 42 percent were single, 32 percent engaged, 24 percent were married, and 2 percent divorced, widowed, or separated. All the married girls resided in the rural areas and only unmarried or engaged girls were interviewed in the towns. Married adolescents in the urban areas were sufficiently rare that it would have greatly increased the time and economic costs of the study to include them in the sample. Of particular note are the extremely low levels of female education. In rural areas only 2 percent of girls were currently in school compared with 40 percent of their urban counterparts. The figures for school enrollment at the time of the survey were 10 percent for rural boys and 66 percent for urban boys.

Of all the adolescents interviewed, 44 percent of the boys and 69 percent of the girls admitted ever having had sex. The relatively higher proportion of girls who said they had had intercourse reflects the high percentage who were married or engaged. The majority of the sample was composed of people of Bambara ethnic origin. It will be discussed below that among the Bambara, marriage tends to be a process with a man obtaining sexual rights and access to a girl once a formal engagement has been consolidated between their two families with a ceremonial exchange of kola nuts. Thus, premarital sexual activity is relatively difficult to define as large numbers of engaged girls may be having sexual relations with their fiances, and even bear them children, before being formally married. In addition, although premarital virginity is technically valued, sexual relations before marriage with someone other than the future husband does occur despite not being condoned culturally. Once married, however, women are required to be faithful to their husbands with a strong social condemnation of those who indulge in extramarital affairs. By contrast, for men, premarital sexual activity is generally socially acceptable, and, after marriage, the institutions of polygyny and "deuxième bureau" contribute to the availability of multiple sexual partners. Of those who had ever had sex, 76 percent of boys and 93 percent of girls admitted to having had sex in the last year. The fact that approximately one-quarter of boys who had ever had intercourse in their lives had not had sex in the last twelve months reflects the somewhat sporadic nature of unmarried adolescents' sexual relations reported elsewhere in the literature (Bohmer and Kirumira 1997). Girls' more regular sexual relations again reflects the high proportions who are married or engaged.

ECONOMIC EXCHANGES AFTER SEXUAL RELATIONS

For those who had ever been sexually active, a sexual history was taken of their encounters over the last year. They were asked to describe the nature of their relationship (kin, nonkin) with each partner, the approximate frequency of intercourse, contraceptive use, and their giving or receiving of gifts or cash. Interviewers were asked to confirm with the interviewees that the economic exchanges in question were directly related to sexual relations rather than those of a more general nature.

The mean number of lifetime sexual partners and those over the last year for ever sexually active males and females is shown in Table 9.1. Clearly, among girls, those who are single appear to have had a slightly higher number of partners than those who are married or engaged and, in general, boys have had a greater number of lifetime partners than girls. There were, however, significant differences according to place of residence, particularly for boys, reflecting the lower proportions of married and engaged adolescents in urban areas and the greater sexual freedom they thus enjoy. Urban girls had had a mean number of 1.61 partners in their lifetime compared with 1.27 for rural girls ($F = 23.8$, $df = 1$, $p < 0.001$). Over the last 12 months, urban girls had had 1.28 partners compared with 1.08 for their rural counterparts ($F = 30.9$, $df = 1$, $p < 0.001$). Likewise, urban boys had had a mean number of 3.57 lifetime partners compared with 2.08 for rural boys ($F = 8.7$, $df = 1$, $p < 0.001$). Over the last year, urban boys had had 1.47 partners over the last year compared with 1.03 for rural boys, although this difference was not statistically significant. We recognize however, as observed elsewhere, that boys may tend to overestimate their number of partners and girls to underestimate due to gender-related expectations of male and female sexual behavior (Youn 1996).

Table 9.1
Mean Number of Sexual Partners over the Lifetime and during the last 12 Months (ever sexually active adolescents only)

	Mean Number of Partners	
	Lifetime	Last 12 months
Girls		
Single (N = 175)	1.61	1.28
Engaged (N = 213)	1.34	1.15
Married (N = 222)	1.28	1.06
Boys		
Single (N = 339)	3.13	1.46

Table 9.2 shows the percentage of boys and girls ever and always giving and receiving cash or gifts with any of their sexual partners over the last year. The survey did not ask about the monetary value of the gift or about the exact sum of cash involved. However, informal discussions with adolescents indi-

cated that girls may hope to receive perhaps the equivalent of $1 to $2 in cash, a soft drink, or sauce condiments. Urban girls reported gifts of a higher value including T-shirts, wraparounds (cloth), or hair extensions, particularly around festival days. They, in turn, gave their male partners not only cash but also cigarettes, local tea, or kola nuts (a mild stimulant).

Table 9.2
Percentage of Adolescents Who Have Ever or Always Given and Received Cash or a Gift with Any Partner during the Last 12 Months

	Any Partner				Last Partner			
	% Giving		% Receiving		% Giving		% Receiving	
	Ever	Always	Ever	Always	Ever	Always	Ever	Always
Girls								
Single (N = 162)	62	16	80	35	57	14	67	33
Engaged (N = 205)	51	10	65	28	48	9	64	26
Married (N = 204)	56	7	59	17	54	6	59	16
All Girls (N = 571)	56	11	67	26	53	10	67	25
Boys								
Single (N = 242)	74	23	62	5	70	16	58	3

Table 9.2 indicates that the giving and receiving of cash or gifts is quite sporadic and irregular. Although over half of all respondents reported ever giving and receiving something, the highest proportion always receiving cash or a gift resources after sexual encounters was among single girls (35 percent). It should be noted that "always" may not mean that the respondent gave or received every single time, but reflects the fact that the vast majority of sexual encounters were followed by the giving or receiving of cash or a gift. A similar proportion of single boys (23 percent) reported always giving a gift or cash after sex, regardless of the number of partners they had had in the last year. Notably, higher proportions of married women reported ever receiving a gift or cash when compared with those interviewed during the Mali Demographic and Health Survey (1995-1996). This may be because they included gifts received before marriage when they were their current husband's fiancee or girlfriend when gift giving is more frequent.

Table 9.2 shows that nearly two-thirds of boys reported ever receiving a gift or cash from their female partners while just 5 percent reported that this was always the case. As described above, marriage is a process among this predominantly Bambara sample. Results presented elsewhere have indicated that, in terms of their reproductive behavior and contraceptive use, there is very little difference between engaged and married girls in that both have much lower rates of family planning uptake and higher fertility than single women (Castle, Yaro and Konate 1999). However, Table 9.2 seems to indicate that, in terms of their financial expectations and gains, engaged girls actually resemble single adolescents rather than their married counterparts. Higher proportions of both single and engaged girls reported ever receiving when compared with married women ($\chi^2 = 18.7$, $df = 2$, $p < 0.001$) and higher proportions of single and engaged girls reported always receiving cash or a gift after intercourse ($\chi^2 = 16.71$, $df = 2$, $p < 0.001$).

The same trends are evident for the last sexual partner and indicate, again, that single girls and those who are engaged are more likely to always receive cash or a gift compared with married women. One-third of single girls reported receiving something after every sexual encounter compared with just over one-third of engaged girls and 16 percent of married women ($\chi^2 = 14.67$, $df = 2$, $p < 0.001$). Over twice the percentage of single girls also reported ever giving a gift when compared with married women. Interestingly, further analysis indicated that 13 percent of engaged girls classified their last partner as someone other than their fiance. This further explains why their economic behavior surrounding sexual relations is more like that of single girls than that of married women. Of those engaged girls who had sex with their fiances, a smaller proportion (22 percent) reported always receiving cash or a gift, compared with those engaged girls whose partner was not their future husband (50 percent). Despite the small size of this subsample this difference was statistically significant ($\chi^2 = 9.05$, $df = 1$, $p < 0.01$). Engaged girls may thus be seeking sexual relations with someone other than their fiance and may be doing so precisely because he does not support them financially to the degree that they require.

Over half of all boys reported ever receiving financial recompense from their last partner, but only a very small percentage (3 percent) received something after every sexual encounter. The overall differences in the proportions of boys and girls receiving after every encounter was statistically significant ($\chi^2 = 51.36$, $df = 2$, $p < 0.001$) as was the difference in the proportions giving after each episode of intercourse ($\chi^2 = 6.6$, $df = 1$, $p < 0.05$).

As the proportions of married adolescent girls giving and receiving regularly is fairly small, and as their sexual relations occur within the conjugal setting, which entails different economic expectations and obligations, the rest of the analysis will focus upon the exchanges between single and engaged female adolescents and single boys.

Table 9.3 shows the reciprocity of the giving and receiving between the unmarried adolescents interviewed and their last sexual partner. It indicates that, among boys, there was a fair degree of reciprocity in the giving and receiving. Eighty-nine percent of those who had ever given had also received something from their girlfriend or sexual partner. By contrast, around half of those

Table 9.3
Reciprocity of Giving and Receiving among Unmarried Sexually Active Adolescents and Their Last Sexual Partner

	% Giving	
Whether Received	Ever	Never
Single girls (N = 162)		
Ever	55	66
Never	45	34
Total	100	100
Engaged girls (N = 205)		
Ever	56	32
Never	44	68
Total	100	100
Single boys (N = 242)		
Ever	89	45
Never	11	55
Total	100	100

who had never given had also never received. Among girls, the distribution of giving and receiving was more unequal depending on whether they were single or engaged. Among both groups, around half of those who had ever given had also received cash or a gift at least once from their last partner. However, among engaged girls nearly two-thirds of those who had never given anything to their last partner had also never received anything. By contrast, two-thirds of single girls who had also never given anything to their partner had received something from him at least once in return for sex. The difference in the percentage of engaged and single girls never giving anything and yet receiving a gift or cash reward was statistically significant ($\chi^2 = 10.07$, $df = 1$, $p < 0.01$). This implies that the formalizing of their relationship into an engagement in some ways lessens the obligation of girls to reciprocate if their fiance gives them a gift. Their impending marriage is perhaps perceived by the girl to be more than enough to repay any such gestures made by her future husband as he will soon have complete rights to her labor and reproduction. As described, a fairly considerable proportion (13 percent) of engaged girls reported that their last sexual partner was not their fiance. Interestingly, among those engaged girls whose last partner was their fiance, and to whom they never gave cash or a gift, only 27 percent reported always receiving some kind of financial benefit after sexual relations. By contrast, among those engaged girls whose last partner was not their fiance, 86 percent of those who had not themselves given anything reported always receiving a gift or cash. This implies that a formal engagement lessens the need for financial reciprocation. However, more casual contacts or those with little hope of future consolidation into marriage are recompensed by financial rewards from the man to the woman with little obligation on her part to reciprocate.

In order to investigate this further, the giving of gifts and/or cash was analyzed by each type of partner for the last partner encountered and the results are shown in Table 9.4. Thirty-one boys had had sexual relationships with friends, acquaintances, and "informal" girlfriends. Nearly one-third claimed to have given something on at least one occasion and nearly one-fifth said they always gave to these partners. Similarly, for the fourteen cases where the relationship was with a neighbor, street vendor, domestic worker, or the like, nearly 30 percent of boys claimed to always provide a financial reward. By contrast, relationships with formalized "girlfriends" ("copines") constituted 80 percent of their sexual contacts. Among these, over three-quarters (77 percent) said that they had at some point given cash or a gift. However, the percentage *always* giving to formal girlfriends dropped to just 12 percent, a lesser percentage than that cited for the informal girlfriends and other sporadic partners. This implies that, as the relationship becomes formalized and its duration increases, the need to consolidate it or to continue to attract the partner by cash incentives is lessened. By contrast, those boys whose relationships would never be normally accepted, perhaps because of social class differences between the two parties (such as between the boys and domestic servants), seem to exchange gifts more regularly despite the sporadic nature of the liaison. This may be because social rewards such as potential marriage are deemed impossible, and because the poor economic status of the female partner may make financial rewards the primary goal of her sexual encounter. In addition, Table 9.4 shows that four of the boys had had contact with formal sex workers all of whom they had paid.

Table 9.4
Giving to Last Partner by Type of Relationship

	Fiance	Girlfriend / boyfriend	Acquaintance	Other	Prostitute
Boys					
N	—	193	31	14	4
% ever giving	—	77	32	50	100
% always giving	—	12	19	29	100
Girls					
N	182	180	2	3	—
% ever giving	44	60	100	0	—
% always giving	7	15	—	—	—

Among girls, 49 percent of their last encounters were with their fiances. Of these, Table 9.4 shows that 44 percent gave something to their male partner. By contrast, 49 percent of their encounters were with their formalized boyfriends ("copains"), and of these, 60 percent of the girls had ever given a gift or money. However, the percentage always giving to fiances and formal boyfriends dropped dramatically to 7 percent and 15 percent, respectively. This again implies that, at the beginning of a relationship, giving may serve to consolidate it and retain the interest of the other party. As its duration increases and its public nature becomes evident, the need for cash exchanges decreases. Thus, for both boys and girls, Table 9.4 clearly shows that gifts of cash or kind are given from girls to boys. It also shows that regular giving decreases as the relationship becomes more formalized and increases if the partner is a casual acquaintance.

SOCIOECONOMIC, SEXUAL, AND PSYCHOLOGICAL FACTORS ASSOCIATED WITH GIRLS ALWAYS RECEIVING CASH OR A GIFT AFTER INTERCOURSE

The next sections will look at girls' receipt of cash and/or gifts and at boys' giving of such items because the results presented above clearly show that this is the most common direction of transfer. Although girls do give and boys do receive reimbursements, the occurrence of such events is relatively rare and would compromise the validity of the bivariate and multivariate analyses presented below.

Table 9.5 shows selected socioeconomic variables associated with always receiving some kind of financial benefit after sex. The table indicates that with increasing age, girls seem less likely to receive financial gain. This is likely to be because the probability of their being engaged increases as they get older and, as shown above, fiancees seem less likely to receive gifts from male partners than girlfriends. Formal schooling was associated with a higher proportion of girls receiving gifts. This result is similar to those found during the Demographic and Health Survey (EDS I, 1995-1996) presented above.

The household economic score represents the grouped results of a rotated factor analysis of household possessions using a varimax rotation. It provides, in one variable, a measure of wealth and of urbanization in that the most expensive, and therefore rarest, items, such as a car, television, and refrigerator, are generally found in urban areas. Table 9.5 shows that significantly higher proportions of wealthier, urban girls receive some kind of financial recompense more or less every time they have sex. This is probably because, as described, their partners are likely to be economically better off and more able to provide these economic incentives. Girls were also asked if they were able to control the income they earned or whether they were obliged to give a significant proportion of it away to friends and relatives to whom they were obligated in the social hierarchy. Commonly in Malian society, age and gender hierarchies endow older individuals and men with rights to the economic resources of those obligated to them. Thus, an older brother may ask a younger brother for cash, a mother may ask her daughter to contribute to the household food budget. Those asked, if in an inferior position to the requestor in the institutionalized social hierarchy, are often obliged to give up their earnings, whether or not they want to. There was, however, little difference in the proportions controlling their own income who received cash in exchange for sex when compared with those who were unable to retain what they earned.

Interestingly, the type of relationship (whether it was continuous or stable versus sporadic) also resulted in significantly differing proportions of girls receiving and not receiving cash or gifts. A greater proportion of those in stable relationships (that is to say, where the partner was usually present and where sexual contact was relatively frequent) were more likely to receive. The duration of the relationship had little effect on the proportions receiving financial reimbursement, but the age of the partner was significant. Over one-third more girls with partners ten or more years older than themselves received money or a gift compared with those with partners less than ten years older. This illustrates the "sugar daddy" phenomenon and is consistent with the literature reviewed above from elsewhere in Africa. A higher percentage of those who had other partners in the last year had received cash from their last partner compared with those who had been faithful to the last partner. This may indicate that certain girls actively pursue economic gains through sex, seeking to accumulate multiple partners to maximize their financial benefits.

Table 9.5
Percentage of Unmarried Girls (N = 361) Always Receiving a Gift or Cash after Sexual Relations with Last Partner by Selected Factors (one-night stands removed from analysis)

	% Always Receiving	Significance
Socioeconomic Factors		
Age		
<18	33	
>18	22	$p < 0.05$
Formal schooling		
Yes	33	
No	26	
Household economic score		
High	36	
Low	24	$p < 0.05$
Controls own income		
Yes	30	
No	27	
Type of Relationship		
Stability of relationship		
Stable/continuous	32	
Sporadic	18	$p < 0.05$
Partner is fiance		
Yes	26	
No	33	
Duration of relationship		
More than one year	27	

Continued

	% Always Receiving	Significance
Less than one year	33	
Age of partner		
Ten or more years older	40	
Less than ten years older	28	$p < 0.05$
Other partners in last year		
Yes	37	
No	27	
Sexual Debut		
First intercourse for cash		
Yes	66	
No	26	$p < 0.001$
Age at first intercourse		
10-15 years	36	
16 years +	20	$p < 0.001$
Psychological Characteristics		
Internal locus of control		
Yes	21	
No	33	$p < 0.05$
High assertiveness		
Yes	35	
No	25	$p < 0.05$
High self-esteem		
Yes	24	
No	39	$p < 0.05$

The two most significant variables in Table 9.5 relate to the context of the girl's first intercourse. Two-thirds of those who had their very first sexual encounter for the purpose of obtaining money or a gift received money from their last partner every time they had intercourse, compared with just over one-quarter who had their first intercourse for other reasons, such as love or curiosity or due to peer pressure. Similarly, over one-third of those who had their first intercourse below age sixteen now received cash for sex compared with one-fifth of those who first had sex after age sixteen.

The last three variables presented in Table 9.5 also indicate that there those who do and who do not have sex that is subsequently reimbursed by cash or a gift possibly have different psychological perspectives on the meaning and purpose of intercourse. Measures of self-esteem, assertiveness, and locus of control were calculated from the answers to questions in a locally devised psychological test using standard scoring methods. The exact nature of the instrument and calculation of scores are described in detail elsewhere (Castle et al. 2000). Overall frequencies derived from the scores created from the answers to specific questions that sought to capture each trait were divided into high, medium, and low self-esteem and assertiveness, and into internal, medium, and external locus of control. Those with an internal locus of control feel that they can control what happens to them and have some power over their life and destiny. Those with an external locus of control feel that their lives are dictated by God, chance, or supernatural forces.

All three psychological traits demonstrated a statistically significant relationship with the percentage of girls always receiving cash after sexual relations. Just over one-fifth of those with an internal locus of control received cash after sex compared with one-third of those with an external locus of control. This may be because again those having sex explicitly for financial gain are, it seems, likely to be those who have started to have sex at an earlier age, possibly before they felt ready. Further analysis showed that of those who had their first intercourse at age fifteen or below, 83 percent said that would preferred to have waited until they were older compared with just 17 percent of those who had their first intercourse at age sixteen or above ($\chi^2 = 20.7$, $df = 1$, $p < 0.001$). They may subsequently perceive that they can do little to control what happens to them, particularly in the sexual arena, and associate intercourse with cash procurement rather than satisfying any social, physical, or emotional need.

Those with a high assertiveness score also seemed more likely to receive cash or a gift after sex than those who were less assertive. This is likely to be because they have the skills to insist on the male partner giving them a reward, particularly if they see cash procurement as one of the main reasons for having sex. However, those with a high self-esteem score comprised lower proportions of those gaining economic benefits after intercourse. Nearly one-quarter of those with high self-esteem gained money or a gift after intercourse compared with over a third with low self-esteem. Again, the latter group may feel devalued and lack self-worth or self-respect if they perceive that one of their main methods of cash procurement is through sex; further qualitative work would need to confirm this.

MULTIVARIATE ANALYSIS OF GIRLS ALWAYS RECEIVING CASH AFTER INTERCOURSE

Table 9.6 presents the results of a logistic regression of the factors presented in Table 9.5 that were associated with receiving cash after every episode of sexual intercourse. The variable "first sex for cash" was, however, eliminated from the analyses as it was highly associated not only with the dependent variable but also with "number of other partners," particularly for those who had only ever had one sexual partner. Table 9.6 shows that, in general, the statistically significant relationships that were evident from the bivariate analysis held when controlling for other factors such as age and education in the multivariate analysis. Table 9.6 clearly shows that the factors exhibiting the strongest associations with girls receiving cash for sex were those relating to their wealth, the type of relationship, their age at first intercourse, and their psychological characteristics. If a girl came from a wealthy household (according to the composite possessions' index created by the factor analysis), she was approximately twice as likely to receive cash after every sexual encounter when compared with girls from poorer households. As described, girls from higher-income families may attract higher-income partners who are better able to compensate them.

Girls with partners ten or more years older than themselves (the "sugar daddy" effect) were 1.80 times more likely to be rewarded after intercourse than girls with younger partners although this association is borderline in terms of its statistical significance ($p = 0.06$). Girls who had their first intercourse at age fifteen or below were 2.10 times more likely to have received cash from their last sexual partner when compared with those whose first intercourse was at age sixteen and above. As described, those regularly receiving financial compensation after sexual relations are likely to present a specific psychological profile that is different from those who do not expect or rely upon sex as a means of gaining cash. Table 9.6 indicates that those with an internal locus of control were 54 percent less likely to have received money from their last sexual partner and those with high self-esteem were 50 percent less likely to have done so. Together, the significant "sexual debut" and psychological variables indicate that later behavior, in terms of regularly receiving cash after sex, probably results from early sexual experiences that form and define girls' perceptions about the purpose of intercourse, their perceived ability to control what happens to them, and their ideas concerning the relative importance or efficacy of using sex versus other methods (such as small enterprise or business activities, for example) to procure cash.

Table 9.6
Multivariate Analysis of Always Receiving Cash after Intercourse with Last Partner (unmarried girls, N = 339)

Variable	Odds Ratio	Significance	Confidence Interval
Socioeconomic Factors			
Age	0.87		0.68–1.09
Formal school	1.41		0.73–2.72
Wealthy	2.06	**	1.14–3.71
Controls own cash	1.02		0.59–1.76
Type of Relationship			
Stable/continuous	2.12	*	1.03–4.36
Partner is fiance	0.76		0.40–1.45
Lasted over a year	0.75		0.42–1.35
Partner is 10+ years older	1.80		0.97–3.36
Other partners in last year	1.39		0.71–2.70

Continued

Variable	Odds Ratio	Significance	Confidence Interval
Sexual Debut			
First intercourse < age 16	2.10	*	1.15–3.82
Psychological Characteristics			
Internal locus of control	0.46	**	0.25–0.81
High self-esteem	0.50	*	0.29–0.84
High assertiveness	1.43		0.57–2.38

*$p < 0.05$; **$p < 0.01$.

SOCIOECONOMIC, SEXUAL, AND PSYCHOLOGICAL FACTORS ASSOCIATED WITH BOYS ALWAYS GIVING CASH OR A GIFT AFTER INTERCOURSE

Table 9.7 shows the percentage of boys giving a gift or money to their last partner after more or less every sexual encounter. It indicates that the age of the partner and age at first intercourse appear significantly associated with this phenomenon. As for the girls' bivariate analyses of factors associated with receiving cash, schooling and high household wealth appeared to be associated with boys giving such rewards although the association was not statistically significant. The association was statistically significant, with those boys who controlled most of their income being 66 percent less likely to give. Indeed, boys' replying that they were unable to hold on to their cash may in fact be relinquishing control to their sexual partners. It seems that it may be the girls' ability to demand cash rather than boys' willingness to exchange it spontaneously that drives these transactions. Girls' ability to demand cash is perhaps linked to their psychological characteristics, and they are able to request or insist upon financial recompense after sex.

Those boys who were in a more sporadic relationship appeared more likely to give every time. Interestingly, this is not consistent with the girls' table, which indicated that female adolescents were more likely to receive from partners with whom they had a stable relationship. The differences may be attributable to variations in the definition of "stable" between boys and girls with girls tending to overreport that their boyfriends were stable or regular partners. Those in a relationship of over one year's duration were more likely to receive every time, while those who had partners younger than themselves were more likely to give than those who had partners of the same age or older. There was little difference in the percentage of boys giving by the number of partners over the last year, suggesting that the amounts given may be fairly small so as not to impede giving to multiple partners.

As for the girls, a highly significant association occurred between boys' age at first intercourse and the proportion engaging in a regular cash transfer after sex. One-quarter of those who had had their first intercourse at age fifteen or below had given cash to their last partner after each sexual encounter compared with just 11 percent of those who had their first sexual experience at sixteen years of age or above. This again implies that early intercourse occurs in a context where cash for sex is more frequent and acceptable, and suggests that those providing financial incentives later on in life may be part of a subgroup with different views about the meaning and purpose of sexual relations. Such boys may also have a different psychological outlook, leading them to think of sex as something that can be bought, rather than as something that occurs in a relationship with broader social and emotional implications and obligations. Table 9.7 shows, for example, that a greater percentage of those with low self–esteem regularly gave cash or a gift in exchange for sex, although, unlike the girls' results presented in Table 9.5, none of the psychological variables were statistically significant.

Table 9.7
Percentage of Unmarried Boys (N = 203) Always Giving a Gift or Cash after Sexual Relations with Last Partner by Selected Socioeconomic Factors (one night-stands removed from the analysis)

	% Always Giving	Significance
Socioeconomic Factors		
Age		
<18	11	
>18	17	
Formal schooling		
Yes	17	
No	11	
Household economic score		
High	19	
Low	11	
Controls own income		
Yes	9	
No	19	
Type of Relationship		
Stability of relationship		
Stable/continuous	10	
Sporadic	22	$p < 0.05$
Partner is girlfriend		
Yes	13	
No	33	$p < 0.05$
Duration of relationship		
More than one year	21	
Less than one year	14	
Age of partner		
Younger	18	
Same age or older	9	

Continued

	% Always Giving	Significance
Other partners in last year		
Yes	18	
No	12	
Sexual Debut		
Age at first intercourse		
10-15 years	25	
16 years +	8	$p < 0.01$
Psychological Characteristics		
Internal locus of control		
Yes	15	
No	14	
High assertiveness		
Yes	15	
No	8	
High self-esteem		
Yes	12	
No	16	

Table 9.8
Multivariate Analysis of Always Giving Cash after Intercourse with Last Partner (unmarried boys, N = 203)

Variable	Odds Ratio	Significance	Confidence Interval
Socioeconomic Factors			
Age	1.07		0.68–1.68
Formal school	1.87		0.55–6.33
Wealthy	1.68		0.58–5.90
Controls own cash	0.34	*	0.12–0.95
Type of Relationship			
Stable/continuous	0.51		0.20–1.31
Lasted over a year	2.21		0.84–5.80
Partner is younger	3.76	*	1.21–11.65
Other partners in last year	1.63		0.64–4.14
Sexual Debut			
First intercourse < age 16	2.89	*	1.13–7.35

Continued

Variable	Odds Ratio	Significance	Confidence Interval
Psychological Characteristics			
Internal locus of control	0.94		0.34–2.59
High self-esteem	0.55		0.20–1.47
High assertiveness	0.35		0.34–3.55

*$p < 0.05$.

MULTIVARIATE ANALYSIS OF BOYS ALWAYS GIVING CASH AFTER INTERCOURSE

Table 9.8 shows that, as for the girls, the association of age at first intercourse with current giving of cash or gifts to the last partner holds when controlling for other socioeconomic and demographic factors. Those boys who first experienced sexual intercourse at age fifteen or below were 2.9 times more likely to give money or a present to their last sexual partner. Other statistically significant results include the fact that boys who are able to control their own cash are 77 percent less likely to give, and those with a partner the same age or younger than themselves are 66 percent less likely to financially reimburse her after each sexual encounter, again perhaps because older partners are able to be more assertive and demanding. Unlike for the girls, the psychological factors do not exert a statistically significant impact on the likelihood of giving.

As suggested above, Tables 9.6 and 9.8 together imply that it is perhaps the girl's ability to procure a gift or to insist on reimbursement that results in the transaction rather than the boy's voluntarily offering some form of compensation without being asked. The importance of the psychological factors for girls in Table 9.6, in combination with the fact that it is boys who are unable to hold on to their cash who are significantly more likely to give financial rewards after sex, implies that the reason they are unable to keep hold of their income is because their female partners are sufficiently assertive to relieve them of it. However, further research, preferably of a qualitative, longitudinal nature, is needed to confirm this hypothesis.

In addition, the results presented here point to a subgroup of adolescent girls who start to have intercourse at a very early age for reasons different from those of the general population. For this group, cash transactions become an integral part of sexual relations. Table 9.9 indicates that a higher proportion of those girls who had their first sex at under age sixteen, had had their first sex for cash (11 percent) compared with those whose first sex was after age sixteen (5 percent). Table 9.9 also shows that economic necessity may have precipitated the girls' early sexual debut as a greater proportion of those delaying their first intercourse were from wealthier households. In addition, one-quarter of those who had sex at an earlier age would have preferred to have waited until they were older compared with just 7 percent of those who started to have intercourse at age sixteen or above. This may indicate that early sex was under forced circumstances. Most significantly, 39 percent of those who had sex below age sixteen now always received cash from the last partner compared with 20 percent of those who had sex at a later age.

The variables presented in Table 9.9 imply that there is a typology of adolescent girl whose first sexual experience (at an early age and for money) shapes the rest of her sexual life, with the result that the majority of her subsequent sexual encounters are accompanied, or even driven, by financial gain. The roots of these behaviors are likely to lie in the poverty and powerlessness that many girls live through and in the fact that gender relations are such that men can provide an immediate and long-term solution to financial problems by reimbursing sexual favors with cash. However, the relationship with poverty is unclear as both Table 9.5 and Table 9.6 indicated that it is, in fact, adolescents from richer households who exchange cash for sex most regularly. Girls from richer households are likely to attract richer partners who can recompense them more regularly. Among these girls, it is more likely that there is a particular group of psychological factors that structure this subgroup's gender relations so that, as time goes on, they perhaps make less of a distinction between economic transactions and sexual needs.

Table 9.9
Correlates of Age at First Intercourse for Girls

	Age at first intercourse		
	Below age 16	Above age 16	
% from wealthy households	39	52	$p < 0.01$
% who would have preferred to delay first sex	11	5	$p < 0.05$
% having first sex for cash	25	7	$p < 0.001$
% now always receiving cash from last partner	39	30	$p < 0.001$

THE CONTEXT OF ECONOMIC EXCHANGES: EVIDENCE FROM THE QUALITATIVE DATA

A principal theme to emerge from the focus group discussions with girls about their reasons for intercourse was the economic benefits they received in exchange for sex. An increasingly materialistic world combined with intensive media exposure appears to be changing adolescents' aspirations, and as the demand for modern, sophisticated fashion or household items increases, girls seem to frequently see intercourse as a means to gaining cash to purchase them.

In particular, some girls appear to engage in sexual activity for the first time to achieve their economic ends.

(Economic) ambition pushes certain girls in Douentza to have their first sexual relations to earn money without being prepared or even wanting it.

[Focus group, uneducated unmarried girls, Douentza (urban)]

Often young women aspire to a lot of things, but they don't have the means (to buy them). So they give themselves unwittingly to men without being ready.

[Focus group, uneducated married girls, Kolokani (rural)]

This phenomenon was much more apparent in urban areas where education and exposure to the modern world—for example, through television—has given girls material aspirations that they can sometimes only meet through sexual activity.

There has been a change because even here at school my classmates encourage each other to act "loose" by showing them the money that they get from their lovers. So certain ones are driven to imitate their classmates; that is to say, they themselves find lovers and begin to have sex before being married.

[Focus group, educated unmarried girls, Douentza (urban)]

Young girls today are ambitious. They take money from men to satisfy their needs. They are obliged to have sex to pay for the things they want because they have to have absolutely everything that their friends have.

[Focus group, uneducated married girls, Douentza (urban)]

Boys saw girls as dominating the sexual arena, particularly in urban areas, and accused them of inciting them to have intercourse when they were, in fact, unwilling. However, it may be that this proactive stance described as characterizing the girls is because they see the potential financial advantages of having sex.

Changing family responsibilities for the economic needs of adolescent girls appears to drive them to engaging in sex for cash. Other focus group data presented above, as well as evidence from elsewhere in West Africa (Delaunay 1994), has seen a rise in individualism resulting in young people choosing their own spouses, rather than leaving the arrangements to their families. The same phenomenon seem to be occurring with regard to economic responsibilities, with young people, particularly in urban areas, being required to be financially independent rather than relying on family support.

The situation has changed because beforehand parents paid for all the expenses of their children, but now there are girls who have to take on all their own expenses and that's why they have to have sex before marriage.

[Focus group, educated unmarried girls, Douentza (urban)]

It's true that children don't listen to their parents any more but I think that the reason is that the parents don't satisfy the (economic) needs of their children so girls do what they have to in order to get money to provide for themselves.

[Focus group, uneducated married girls, Douentza (urban)]

Table 9.10
Reproductive Risk among Boys who Always and Sometimes Gave Money to Last Sexual Partner

	Always gave	Sometimes/ Never gave	Ever gave	Never gave
N	38	204	71	167
Partner change				
Mean number of lifetime partners	3.55	3.05	3.31	2.72
Mean number of partners in last year	1.45	1.46	1.47	1.43
% with at least one partner at time of survey	68	70	77	54
% with more than one partner at time of survey	18	9	11	11
Contraceptive use				
% ever used modern method	58	37	42	36
% ever used condom	58	36	41	36
% using condom with last partner	13	15	15	13

REPRODUCTIVE HEALTH RISKS AND THE ECONOMIC CONTEXT OF SEXUAL RELATIONS

Table 9.10 shows the reproductive health risk incurred by boys who always and sometimes gave cash or a gift to their last sexual partner. It indicates that, as suggested by the preceding analyses, those who always give some kind of reimbursement exhibit significantly higher risk behaviors than those who sometimes or never give. Table 9.10 indicates that those who always gave had a higher number of lifetime partners than those who sometimes or never gave, although this difference was not statistically significant. There was no significant difference in their number of partners over the last twelve months. The percentage of those who always give cash or a gift who had more than one concurrent partner was twice as high compared with those who sometimes or never gave, although due to the small numbers the difference was not statistically significant. Among those who had ever given, a significantly higher proportion had at least one partner at the time of the survey (77 percent) compared with those who had never given (54 percent). This result was statistically significant ($\chi^2 = 11.94$, $df = 1$, $p < 0.001$). It is probably the fact that these boys give cash rewards regularly which makes them more attractive as sexual partners to girls. Those who never give appear to have a higher probability of being sexually abstinent despite having had sexual relations in the past. This is likely to be because they have difficulty in getting a partner if it is widely known that they do not reimburse sexual encounters with material benefits.

Differences were also evident in the contraceptive behavior among those who always, sometimes, and never gave. Table 9.10 shows that a much higher percentage of those who always gave had ever used a modern method of contraception, usually a condom ($\chi^2 = 6.56$, $df = 1$, $p < 0.05$). This is probably because their choice of partners included those with whom they have an informal, nonpublic relationship (neighbors, acquaintances, etc.) and who they may consider high-risk compared with their formal girlfriends with whom they have no need or inclination to give money regularly. There was, however, little difference in the use of condoms during their last sexual encounter by always or sometimes giving cash.

Table 9.11 shows some even more striking differences in the sexual behavior of girls who always, ever, and never received cash for sex. The mean number of lifetime partners among those who always received a financial reward (1.62) was significantly higher than the number for those who sometimes and never received (1.39) ($F = 4.78$, $df = 1$, $p < 0.05$). The mean number of sexual partners over the last year was also smaller for those who never received compared with those who had ever received from their past sexual partner ($F = 7.02$, $df = 1$, $p < 0.01$). This points to the fact that girls who regularly receive money after sex may seek to maximize their number of partners to increase their financial benefits. Alternatively, they may leave certain partners if the latter do not give as much or as regularly as they desire, leading to a higher turnover of partners for those girls who expect or need cash after sex. There was no real difference in the percentage of girls who had at least one partner at the time of the survey by whether they had ever they received cash after intercourse. Unlike the boys, the vast majority of girls had at least one current partner whether they received cash regularly from him or not.

There was, however, a significant difference in the percentage of girls who had more than one partner at the time of the survey by whether they received cash or not from the last partner. Thirteen percent of girls who always received cash from the last partner had at least one other partner compared with just 4 percent of those who only sometimes or never received money or a gift ($\chi^2 = 11.94$, $df = 1$, $p < 0.001$). Again, this implies that some girls have a deliberate strategy of maximizing the number of partners with an aim of getting as much financial support as possible. Of those who had more than one partner (N = 14), and where the last partner always gave a gift, 85 percent of their second partners also always gave a gift while 7 percent gave sometimes, and a further 7 percent not at all. This indicates that rather than girls seeking additional partners because one does not meet their financial needs, they seek to accumulate several partners, the majority of whom give most of the time, in order to maximize their financial advantage from sex.

Table 9.11
Reproductive Risk among Unmarried Girls Who Always and Sometimes Received Money from Their Last Sexual Partner

	Always received	Sometimes/ Never received	Ever received	Never received
N	107	260	261	106
Partner change				
Mean number of lifetime partners	1.62	1.39	1.50	1.36
Mean number of partners in last year	1.30	1.17	1.25	1.10
% with at least one partner at time of survey	97	97	98	94
% with more than one partner at time of survey	13	4	8	2
Contraceptive use				
% ever used modern method	27	20	27	9
% ever used condom	16	12	17	4
% using condom with last partner	13	8	13	1

Concerning contraceptive use, significant differences were evident between those who ever and never received. Three times the percentage of those who had ever received cash or a gift had ever used a modern method of contraception compared with those who had never received ($\chi^2 = 14.31$, $df = 1$, $p < 0.001$). Similarly, a much greater percentage had ever used a condom ($\chi^2 = 10.89$, $df = 1$, $p < 0.001$) and had used a condom with the last partner ($\chi^2 = 12.7$, $df = 1$, $p < 0.001$). There was little difference between the contraceptive behavior of those who always received and those who sometimes or never received. A likely explanation for the fact that those who ever received cash or a gift are more likely to use contraception is that those who never receive are probably fiances or formal girlfriends who may actively seek to become pregnant to consolidate their relationship into marriage. Those in more informal or marginal relationships may try to avoid pregnancy as premarital or preengagement childbearing is socially stigmatized in Bambara society, as described above. It seems that pregnancy rather than STD prevention was the aim of girls' contraceptive use given the high percentage of methods other than the condom that were employed.

CONCLUSION

The study presented here comprises new and original findings concerning the exchange of financial resources after sexual relations among adolescent boys and girls in rural and urban Mali. The data indicate that financial transactions following intercourse are extremely frequent and characterize the majority of sexual encounters. The rates of those giving and receiving cash or gifts among those interviewed during this survey are higher than those found during the Demographic and Health Survey of Mali (EDS, 1995-1996) and than those cited from other studies in West Africa. This may be because interviewers were carefully trained to sensitively probe about this issue and because interviewees were asked about all financial transactions, not just those occurring with the main sexual partner.

The results also showed that transactions do not only occur from boys to girls, but also that the majority of unmarried girls have, at some point, given a gift or cash to their sexual partner following intercourse. For both boys and girls, however, the frequency and regularity of the giving appear to depend on the perceived nature of the relationship and on the age of the partner. In addition, reciprocity among girls and their sexual partners seemed to be associated with whether they perceived that the relationship was going to develop into marriage. Those who were given gifts by their fiances felt no need to reciprocate, while those who classified their partners as boyfriends exchanged gifts or cash more frequently. Boys tended to give more often to those with whom they had sporadic, informally defined, or nonpublic relationships rather than to those whom they classified as formal girlfriends or fiancees.

For girls, the receiving of gifts or cash appeared to be strongly associated with being economically well off, having an older partner, having had their first sexual experience because they wanted money or a gift having had their first intercourse below age sixteen, having an internal locus of control, and exhibiting low self-esteem. For boys, regular giving was done by those who had little control over their income, those whose partners were younger than themselves, and those who also had an early age at first intercourse. The findings suggest that, especially among girls, there is a subgroup of vulnerable individuals whose later economic behavior with regard to sexual relations is instilled in them early on, as their first sexual encounters were motivated by primarily financial reasons.

Boys who give cash and those girls who regularly receive a reward after sexual intercourse exhibit sexual behaviors that put them at a higher risk of catching and transmitting STDs and HIV than the general population. Boys who had ever given a gift had a greater average number of concurrent sexual partners. However, those who always gave a gift were more likely to use condoms than those who never gave or than those who gave irregularly. Among girls, those who always received money or a present from their last partner had a significantly higher average number of sexual partners than those who rarely or never received any kind of recompense. It may not always be the partners' willingness to give that determines girls' rate of partner change, as even those with multiple concurrent partners whose last partners gave them something after each encounter also received some kind of reward the majority of the time from their second partner. The quantitative study did not collect information about the monetary value of the gifts involved, and it may be that girls who receive gifts of low value seek additional recompense elsewhere. A greater proportion of girls who always, or sometimes, received gifts had used a modern method of contraception. In particular, they seemed more likely to use a condom, indicating that they were perhaps aware of their own high-risk behavior and of the background and nature of the partners from whom they were soliciting or receiving financial rewards.

The study raises several important policy implications. First, much of the rhetoric and practical interventions associated with halting the spread of STDs/HIV in sub-Saharan Africa has concentrated on the role of formal and informal prostitution, that is to say, women who admit that their principal source of income is earned in exchange for sex. However, this study indicates that financial transactions after sexual encounters are the norm among female adolescents who would never describe themselves as sex workers. Second, the fact that girls also give financial recompense to boys is also ignored by current research into the motivations and benefits behind adolescent sexual behaviour. Thus, interventions aimed at encouraging low-risk behaviors need to take into account that the current definition of, and focus upon, "prostitutes" is inappropriate in societies where the majority of sexual encounters have a financial dimension and where reciprocal exchanges occur between boys and girls. The results presented here also imply that, in order to reduce financial incentives for sex, particularly among young girls, it is necessary to replace the economic gains they receive from intercourse with opportunities to gain income from other nonsexual sources such as microenterprise or credit programs. The research also clearly shows that the psychological forces driving young people to equate sexual relations with financial gain are formed early in their sexual careers. Thus, interventions need to focus upon the very young, and even on those who have yet to start to be sexually active, in order to make them aware of the risks involved and of other opportunities to gain regular income besides sex.

This study begs as many questions as it answers and highlights the need for further work to: first, identify exactly when ideas about the purpose and motivations for sexual intercourse are formed; second, target individuals at an early age who exhibit an elevated risk of engaging in sex for financial reasons; and, third, identify possible alternatives, particularly for girls, to relying primarily on sex as a means of accruing financial advantage. Longitudinal, qualitative research could shed light on the evolution of high-risk behaviors and financial expectations and inform program managers and policymakers as to how to give economically viable alternatives to young people while ensuring that they have safe, risk-free sexual lives.

NOTE

The authors gratefully acknowledge the helpful advice of Mohamadou Gueye and Dennis Ahlberg with the multivariate analyses. Funding for the study was provided by the Rockefeller Foundation.

REFERENCES

Ankomah, A. (1996). Premarital relationships and livelihood in Ghana. *Gender and Development* 4(3): 39–47.

Aryee, A. (1997). The African family and changing nuptiality patterns. Pp. 78–96 in A. Adepoju (ed.). *Family, Population and Development in Africa.* London: Zed.

Bohmer, L., and E. Kirumira. (1997). *Access to Reproductive Health Services; Participatory Research with Ugandan Adolescents.* Makrere University, Child Development Centre/Pacific Institute for Women's Health. Los Angeles: Pacific Institute for Women's Health.

Carael, M., J. Cleland, and R. Ingham. (1994). Extra-marital sex: Implications for survey results for STD/HIV transmission. *Health Transition Review.* 4, Supplement: 153–172.

Castle, S., Y. Yaro, and M. Konate. (1999). Links between psychological factors, status and sexual behaviour among Malian adolescents. Paper presented at the Annual Meeting of the Population Association of America, New York.

Coulibaly, S., F. Dicko, S.M. Traoré, S. Sidibe, M. Seroussi, and B. Barrère. (1996). *Enquête Démographique et de Santé, Mali 1995–6.* Calverton, MD: Cellule de Planification et de Statistique du Ministere de la Santé, Direction Nationale de la Statistique et de l'Information et Macro International Inc.

Delaunay V. (1994). *L'entree en vie feconde: Expression demographique des mutations socio-economiques d'un milieu rural senegalais.* Paris, France. Centre Francais sur la Population et le Developpement [CEPED]. 326p. Les Etudes du CEPED No. 7

Finger, W. (1993). Seeking better ways to teach youth about AIDS. *Network* 14(2): 16–19.

Helitzer-Allen, D., and M. Makhambera. (1993). How can we help adolescents avoid HIV infection? *Network* 13(4): 7.

Mati, J. (1989). A review of adolescent health. *Journal of Obstetrics and Gynaecology of Eastern and Central Africa* 8(1): 19–23.

Meekers, D., and G. Ahmed. (1997). Adolescent sexuality in southern Africa: Cultural norms and contemporary behaviour. Population Services International Research Division Working Paper No 2. Washington DC: Population Services International.

Meekers, D., and A-E. Calves. (1996). Main girlfriends, marriage and money; playing the field in sub-Saharan Africa. Population Research Institute Working Paper AD96-02. University Park: Pennsylvania State University.

Nzyuko, S., P. Lurie, W. McFarland, W. Leyden, D. Nyamwaya, and J. Mandel. (1997). Adolescent sexual behaviour along the Trans-Africa highway in Kenya. *AIDS* 11, Supplement 1: S21–26.

Plan International, Mali (1997). *Enquête CAP dans la Region de Sikasso*: Rapport d'analyse. Bamako: Plan International.

Preston-White E. (1996). Survival sex or the culture of sex work in South Africa. *AIDS Bulletin* 5(1): 8–9.

Youn, G. (1996). Sexual activities and attitudes of adolescent Koreans. *Archives of Sexual Behavior* 25(6): 629–643.

10

NEW LIGHT ON THE SUB-SAHARAN AFRICAN FERTILITY TRANSITION: CONCLUSION

John C. Caldwell and Pat Caldwell

This chapter comprises an overview of the evidence presented in the preceding chapters of this book. The attempt will be made to identify the main discoveries and to place them in the context of regional changes and especially regional fertility decline.

The world fertility decline began in France in the late eighteenth century and was evident in most Western countries in the late nineteenth century, spreading to Latin America, Asia, and North Africa from the 1960s. The fundamental cause was massive social and economic change. Indeed, the demographic transition, embodying huge mortality and fertility reductions, can be regarded as the major social dimension of the Industrial Revolution. Mortality decline resulted from rising standards of living, changes of lifestyle associated with the full development of a market economy, and education, together with public health and biomedical breakthroughs. Fertility decline was driven both by these forces and by the mortality transition, especially the greater chance that babies would survive to live to adulthood. Both the mortality and fertility transitions engendered social and political philosophies that regarded them as being desirable and organized movements that promoted their acceleration.

Demographic transition came late to sub-Saharan Africa. By the early 1950s life expectancy was still less than 37 years and the infant mortality rate close to 200 deaths per thousand live births (United Nations 1999). Yet clearly mortality was falling because a total fertility rate of 6.5 implied that life expectancy had earlier (perhaps until the end of the nineteenth century) been less than 25 years. Over the next 30 years life expectancy rose steadily to around 48 years, gaining almost 0.4 years per elapsed year, somewhat slower than the average for the developing world but quite respectable given the ecological conditions of much of the continent. But since the mid-1980s advance against mortality has almost halted, in some countries because of the AIDS epidemic and nearly everywhere because of a slowdown in economic growth. According to Maddison (1995, 1999), the annual average increase in real per capita income between 1950 and 1973 was 2.2 percent in Africa, compared with 2.9 percent for the world, but between 1973 and 1997 it was 0.05 percent compared with 1.3 percent. The stagnation in economic growth doubtless constrained the advance against mortality, but the solutions imposed by structural adjustment programs, with cost recovery for health services, had their own specific impact.

By the early 1950s mortality levels had declined sufficiently to allow an annual population growth rate for the whole of sub-Saharan Africa around 2 percent and by 1980 this was approaching 3 percent. After 1970 fertility decline characterized most parts of the world, but not sub-Saharan Africa. Indeed the United Nations (1999, p. 18) postulates that the total fertility rate slowly rose until about 1970 as the duration of lactation and postpartum abstinence shortened. Thereafter, for the best part of two decades it changed little. We now know that South Africa's fertility probably fell from about 1965 (Caldwell and Caldwell 1993), but its population constituted only 8 percent of the region's.

There has been debate over why sub-Saharan Africa alone failed to achieve fertility decline. The region was poor but, by the early 1980s, India, with a lower real per capita income than Côte d'Ivoire, Ghana, Nigeria, or Kenya, had achieved a fertility decline of 25 percent, and fertility was falling also in Bangladesh with little more than half the real per capita income of these African countries (Maddison 1995; United Nations 1999). And higher African mortality was not the explanation, for the infant mortality rate was higher in India and Bangladesh than in any of the four African countries and life expectancy was similar.

We have suggested a range of reasons for the sustaining of high fertility in sub-Saharan Africa (Caldwell and Caldwell 1987). Traditional culture and religion, faced by the potential for horrific levels of mortality, had strongly supported high fertility and regarded attempts to control it as deeply suspect. Childlessness was abhorred. Children were supported by the extended family, and high levels of fostering, usually by relatives, weakened the connection between biological parentage and economic burden. Land was communally owned and high fertility ultimately increased access to land. Children were an investment for old age guaranteed, at least for their fathers, by strong cultural and religious proscriptions against those who might forget who gave them life. At the national level there were no traditional elites as in Asia ready to provide political and moral leadership in the control of fertility. Indeed, the governments in these new countries have been notably reluctant to provide strong, outspoken leadership in such areas as controlling fertility or combating AIDS. They fear failure, unsure that controlling fertility is the African way and aware that powerful forces such as the Catholic Church are critical. In some places, such as Kenya and Ghana, national family planning programs came into existence almost as early as the Asian programs, but the African bureaucrats have guarded against failure and have not identified as closely with the programs' success as have their Asian counterparts, nor have they produced such efficient systems. Only in apartheid South Africa was a fully efficient contraceptive delivery system organized and that resulted in substantial fertility declines among the black African population. But, because of the racial divide, the South African government and bureaucracy could not provide the active leadership, and even goading, found in Asia. Nevertheless, the South African experience is important because it revealed quite different patterns of contraceptive use between the races. Among black South Africans the demand was for hormonal methods, especially injectables and the pill, while there was only a small demand for intrauterine devices (IUDs) and female sterilization and none for male sterilization. The pattern further north will probably be similar, although IUDs and female sterilization may have a larger role.

We have been skeptical of the organization of African family planning efforts along the female-centered, clinic-centered pattern of Asia (Caldwell and Caldwell 2001). In Asia almost all fertility control was within marriage and most of it was aimed at halting family building. The services were for married women (except the early Indian vasectomy program). In sub-Saharan Africa the need so far has been dominated by a demand for contraception to replace sexual abstinence in the postpartum period, thus maintaining or even extending traditional birth intervals. Contraception has also been in demand for premarital and extramarital relations, the former among young women anxious to complete their education or to establish themselves in a job in the modern economy, and the latter to hide evidence of adulterous relationships or to avoid HIV infection. In a situation where half the demand may come from unmarried women, married women who wish to break with the postpartum abstinence tradition, or men, none of whom want to be seen at the local family planning clinic, there has been a demand for anonymous outside services, shown by the premium many people are willing to pay for commercial services. These services are likely to be constrained by the difficulty small medical stores face in getting contraceptive supplies, or even by legal restrictions on what they can sell.

By the 1990s it was apparent that a fertility transition had begun in most of southern Africa (South Africa, Zimbabwe, Botswana, Namibia, Lesotho, and Swaziland) and Kenya. Recent analysis of small-area data, mostly from the DHS (Demographic and Health Survey) program (Tabutin and Schoumaker 2001), has shown that fertility decline is much more likely to have occurred in large urban centers than in rural areas. Furthermore, the original fertility-transition area, southern Africa, is being joined by others: a stretch of the West African coast comprising Abidjan, Accra, and much of southern Ghana, Lomé, Cotonou, most of southern Nigeria, and Yaoundé/Douala; the Central Province of Kenya; Khartoum and Northern Sudan. Clearly, contraception is being supplemented by abortion. Another analysis (Mahy and Gupta 2001) suggests that women's first birth is being delayed in nearly all urban and many rural areas. It is unclear to what extent delayed marriage is the explanation and to what extent the phenomenon is explained by delayed sexual debut, perhaps associated with a fear of HIV infection.

What is clearer are the factors associated with fertility decline. Tabutin and Schoumaker (2001) showed that the strongest associations with fertility decline were relatively low levels of infant mortality and high levels of two development measures, women's literacy (which can be taken as a proxy for female education), and electrification. The latter might be taken as just a development indicator but for the fact that it has shown up elsewhere in multivariate analyses of fertility decline. It is possible that the arrival of electricity does change ways of life because of the possibility of television, or reading or doing school homework at night, in its making possible small industries, or in inciting the purchase of powered tools or household items. The availability of contraceptives was found to be less important, although Brass and Jolly (1993) reported that in Kenya the closeness of a family planning clinic was of major importance in explaining the level of family planning practice. Even more surprisingly, Tabutin and Schoumaker found that urbanization had no additional effect beyond that of the characteristics of urban population such as education. This seems surprising in view of the greater burden of children in the city with its fully monetized economy, far from supportive rural extended families, and its demand for literacy and education for much of the employment.

The question, then, is to what extent has the research reported in this book sustained or qualified this picture?

THE NEW RESEARCH

The research was carried out in five anglophone countries (Ghana, Kenya, Malawi, Sudan, and Zambia), one francophone one (Mali), and Ethiopia. Four research areas were in countries well advanced in fertility transition (Kenya, Ghana, and Northern Sudan) while the rest still have total fertility rates in the six-to-seven range. The charge that the latter might be unsuited to an inquiry into fertility decline is offset by the fact that three of the studies were confined to urban areas, one reported its main findings from them, and one was in a closely settled, technologically advanced irrigation project.

The research consisted of microstudies only in a specific but valid sense of the term. There were no anthropological studies characterized by long-term residence and community involvement. The closest was the investigation of the Nairobi slums (Dodoo, Sloane, and Zulu) carried out by a qualitative approach, mainly group discussions. Four of the seven studies incorporated focus groups or other group discussions. The aim was usually to provide "thick" description and to elucidate some of the survey responses. Only one investigation, that in Ndola, used focus group discussions to help shape the survey questionnaire. Six of the eight studies included men as well as women. Even more important was the fact that all studies involved original research instruments in contrast to standardized international surveys. Thus the research was tailor-made to investigate each specific topic. Only one, in southern Ghana, incorporated repeated visits to a panel.

The studies, especially those in Mali and Kenya, bring out a point that is important for both family planning and AIDS programs: that the region is characterized by a good deal of premarital and extramarital sexual activity. This has certainly been increased by social change and is probably at its greatest in the towns, but traditional constraints on nonmarital sexual activity have none of the ferocity, especially for females, that is found in most of Asia. This means that both family planning and AIDS programs have to find ways to reach the unmarried. Family planning programs in Asia and North Africa have successfully focused almost exclusively on married women, but to do so in sub-Saharan Africa would constitute a programmatic disaster. The greatest problem is encountered with adolescents. Because both family planning and AIDS programs in sub-Saharan Africa usually operate in an atmosphere of sexual unreality, individual service providers often take an Asian attitude to adolescents seeking services. They are more likely to be prayed over to stop their sinning than to be provided with condoms or other contraceptives. This has been confirmed by every research project that has investigated the matter.

Widespread sexual activity among adolescents, greatest in urban areas, is confirmed by Castle and Konate in Mali, a conservative Sahelien society that is at least 90 percent Muslim. The picture presented in this book and in Gueye et al. (2001) is one where adolescent boys and girls are both pushed by peer pressure to engage in sexual activity, and where their families usually choose to ignore or even condone it. Sex is encouraged by films, television, novels, the new world opened up by schooling, and the rising age at marriage, especially female marriage. Boys undertake sexual escapades largely to validate themselves among their peers. Girls do so often to try to establish or maintain a relationship, but "the focus groups [but not the quantitative survey] were dominated by evidence of [predominantly urban] girls engaging in first and subsequent sex for financial reasons." Girls want both gifts and money, the latter more likely from older male partners, so that they can get clothes and such extras as cosmetics to enjoy a fully modern life. The findings indicate, however, that the direction of transfers is not only from boys to girls, but also that the majority of unmarried girls have, at some point, given a gift or cash to their sexual partner after sexual relations. The frequency and regularity of the giving, for both boys and girls, appears to depend on the perceived nature of the relationship and on the age of the partner. In addition, reciprocity among girls seems to be associated with whether they perceive that the relationship is going to develop into marriage. The findings indicate that indeed in urban areas both girls and boys are largely expected to meet their own expenses as increasing individualism dominates family life.

The authors argue that there exists a subgroup of vulnerable girls whose later economic behavior with regard to sexual relations is instilled in them early on and may entail reproductive health risks. These girls' first sexual encounters (which many had ideally wished to delay) frequently occurred at an early age and were usually motivated by primarily financial reasons. The authors argue for a wider social and economic role for females, which is difficult in a poor, Islamic country where in 1997 fewer than two-fifths of girls were enrolled in primary schools and under one-fifth in secondary schools (but double the proportions of two decades earlier) (World Bank 2001, p. 285). The chapter does not give the impression of a family planning program successfully reaching out to these youngsters even though they live in a society where sexual relations provide for many girls the route out of poverty and a potential way to gain financial security.

A similar, but stronger picture is painted by Dodoo, Sloan, and Zulu of the situation in the Nairobi slums, which house 70 percent of the city's total population. Here, in ethnically mixed rural-urban migrant populations, hanging on in a city where employment is no longer growing, many wholly or partly support themselves by sexual activities. This, apart from beer drinking, which provokes sexual encounters, is one of the few sources of entertainment. The conditions are crowded and sexual activities are often visible. Selling sex is normal. The children see it, but the parents, inhibited by the inability of the society to discuss sexuality across the generation gap, never explain it to them: "the younger members of the community [under fifteen years of age] are socialized, deliberate or otherwise, into thinking that sexual behaviour is normal even for people of their age."

Sex in the slums is a survival strategy. Girls may be sent out to bring back money. Women often dispense with a male partner once he becomes unemployed, and have transactional sex for specific payments that have to be made. Life is lived in an atmosphere created by sex, alcohol, drugs, violence, teenage pregnancies, STDs, and HIV/AIDS. What is striking is that, although everyone knows that they live surrounded by dangerous sex, the discussion groups seem to have said almost nothing about contraceptive use or the activities of family planning or AIDS programs.

Osman provides another insight into social and economic change. This time it is not of the chaos of the Nairobi slums but of an organized settlement in a comparatively new irrigation area in northern Sudan. This is an old Muslim society with characteristics often closer to those of North Africa than sub-Saharan Africa. The organized settlement was a deliberately modernizing experience. There was some employment of women, and child mortality declined because of the provision of health services. Lower child mortality was strongly associated with mother's education and less strongly with higher household income. It seemed the right conditions for the onset of fertility decline. In fact fertility was half a child higher than in surrounding areas and had probably been raised by the project. Part of the explanation was probably that children were hardly a burden, since they had access to free health services and the cotton industry was keen to employ them. More critically, the project did not promote smaller families and its health services did not provide contraception. Clearly, at least in the short term, fertility decline is not a spontaneous reaction to economic development and social change.

In contrast, and only a few hundred kilometers away, Hogan and Berhanu studied a population in rural southern Ethiopia little affected by socioeconomic and demographic modernization. The infant mortality rate was still over 100 per thousand live births, the total fertility rate close to seven, and contraceptive prevalence around 2 percent. Female literacy was under 10 percent, and almost two-thirds of the population believed that the determination of family size was beyond human control. Even in these forbidding circumstances, the researchers found that there was a significant acceptance of contraception when it was offered. This was especially the case where ethnic groups were most mixed, and particularly so among the minority groups (a finding opposed to the long-standing belief that minority status promoted relatively high fertility). Significantly, and supporting the thesis that Asian fertility control has been successful because of reactions to dense populations, contraception was more readily adopted where populations were densest. There may, of course, have been issues of land shortage in such areas. Contraception was also more readily adopted where family levels of literacy and economic activity were highest.

If rural southern Ethiopia is a view of a passing Africa, then urban southern Ghana, researched by Agyei-Mensah, Aase, and Awusabo-Asare, is one of the future. In Accra and Cape Coast socioeconomic change in an urban context has reduced the value of children and increased their cost. In the last three decades the likelihood of assistance from the extended family in meeting these costs has dwindled, and the burden falls almost entirely on the nuclear family. In the elite suburbs parents are concerned about the quality of their children and the quality of their proposed spouses. As a result actual and preferred family size has converged at around three children, with successful family limitation achieved by easily accessible contraception. Marriages are occurring at later ages and even the first birth may be postponed.

In contrast, urban poor women still have the first birth early, either inside or outside marriage, but thereafter practice birth control. In further contrast, fertility in a fishing village is still high even though contraceptive help is accessible. Children in such a village are still of value for earning income and because they are the insurance provision for their parents in time of sickness or old age. Southern Ghanaian urban life is changing, as is evidenced by a total fertility rate in the whole of Greater Accra of 2.7 and in two southern regions of 4.4. The population is, with socioeconomic change, followed by economic adversity, faced with a situation where large families impose unacceptable burdens. In terms of their aims for themselves and their families, these difficulties are most strongly felt by the urban elites, as was the case even forty years ago (Caldwell 1968).

Agyeman and Casterline also worked in southern Ghana, studying organizational membership and employing a panel of individual men and women with six monthly visits. They investigated the level of organizational membership in an effort to explain the diffusion of ideas about fertility control and the means for achieving this end. They also argued that such diffusion would be greater in heterogeneous communities, adding a theoretical dimension to what Hogan and Berhanu had found in southern Ethiopia.

They found that the importance of social organization and heterogeneity in their six study areas have to a very considerable extent been overridden by different community histories with regard to the arrival of family planning knowledge and access. Their different histories in this regard are explained partly by location and partly by happenstance. They concluded that "the stance of political leaders and the effectiveness of health and family planning programs may have substantial bearing on whether transition starts early or late, and whether it proceeds slowly or rapidly," and that the role of family planning workers and exponents is important. Thus much depends on whether there is an effective, penetrating national family planning program.

A later and slower start in the fertility transition has occurred in Malawi and is explored by Zulu and Kalipeni. Indeed modern contraception was banned in Malawi between 1968 and 1984, and the total fertility rate was probably around 7.6 in the early 1980s (United Nations 1999, p. 276). In earlier times the rate was somewhat lower because of postpartum sexual abstinence and other mechanisms for maintaining birth intervals. The chief demand for modern contraception is still to maintain those intervals or even to extend them, as is suggested by a fall in the total fertility rate to 5.6.

When birth intervals were maintained by traditional means, men regarded fertility and its control as being women's business. With the arrival of hormonal methods, men began to want to become involved, partly because they suspected their wives might use these methods to limit family size, and partly because of the suspicion that this would make the wives less cautious about infidelity. The husbands are even more concerned about their wives being sterilized or having abortions without their knowledge and agreement. In reality they are probably frequently left in the dark about abortions, which are reported to be quite common, especially among schoolgirls and lactating married women. Their responses about sterilization are revealing in a subcontinent where male sterilization is virtually nonexistent and female sterilization at a low level. The fear of male sterilization is that it will lead to impotence or an end of manhood in the sense of fertility. We have been inclined to draw a parallel in the case of womanhood, especially given the cultural abhorrence of barrenness. But this research suggests that low levels of female sterilization might arise more from male than female opposition.

The researchers emphasize that it is in relation to the use of modern family planning that husbands feel they should have a greater say about contraception. In the traditional setting the wife was embedded in a network of women, many of them older relations; they look after such women's affairs as reproduction. In the context of modern contraception the husband feels it is now his duty to concern himself with what is going on, but the family planning programs and clinics operate in the style of the Asian prototypes and freeze him out. They assign him no role except as a purchaser of condoms from specific AIDS-oriented condom programs. The authors comment that this is surprising given that sub-Saharan African experimental programs that have been at least partly focused on husbands have been remarkably successful. In the absence of these, husbands are only too likely to be suspicious of family planning programs and all they stand for. Women attending Malawian clinics most favor, as in South Africa, injectables, well suited to birth spacing and also to covert use by the women who wish to control their own bodies and fertility.

The study design employed by Biddlecom and Kaona in Ndoli, in Zambia's Copper Belt, is a model of microfertility research and its findings deserve serious attention. Their central finding is clear: in the somewhat difficult conditions of an African industrial city, around 45 percent of couples use contraception (26 percent modern contraception, mostly hormonal methods), while another 20 percent are classified as exhibiting unmet need. But there are few differences that can be distinguished between the two groups. Often just chance with regard to contraceptive provision separates them. Probably many of the users could, with a small setback, discontinue use, while many of the unmet-need group with a little more discussion or a slightly better service could begin using contraception. An Asian-style program, with the head of state, his ministers, the bureaucracy, and the program all advocating contraception for the good of the country and of the family, could easily raise current use to 60 or 65 percent, consonant with a total fertility rate under three. The problem is not one of poverty or illiteracy but of leadership and organization. The authors say that better programs would warn of and counsel on health side effects and would reach out to men to bring them onside and meet their needs.

Ndola has high levels of STDs and HIV/AIDS. Yet the research convinced its authors that condoms are never going to be used on a significant scale within marriage: nor are premarital or extramarital sexual relations going to disappear. The greatest chance of success is to convince the people, especially the men, that all nonmarital sex has a sufficient element of danger to make it critically important that condoms be used as much as possible, and always in completely commercial relationships. The problem again is most difficult with adolescents. They are the group who find it hardest to ask for condoms and meet the greatest obstacles in being given them. Furthermore, a girl who agrees to sex with a boy in the hope of marrying him finds it difficult to imply that he constitutes a risk of infecting her with STDs and HIV/AIDS.

Once again the researchers found that the family planning services were regarded as being exclusively for women. Three-quarters of the demand for services was for spacing. They also believed abortion to be at quite a high level, mostly sought by schoolgirls and young unmarried women or by married women who had not achieved the desired interval since the last birth. They explain why legal abortions are few, even though Zambia was the first sub-Saharan African country to accept broad socioeconomic conditions for it and still has the most liberal laws outside South Africa. The preliminary procedure is just too cumbersome. The authors seem to hold that these few legal abortions are the only safe ones; this is at odds with evidence from elsewhere in sub-Saharan Africa that the proportion of safe abortions is growing because the number of doctors is increasing and many depend on abortions for much of their income.

THE SITUATION BECOMES CLEARER

Only in the 1990s did it become clear that sub-Saharan Africa was at last joining the global fertility transition. Now we know that it is occurring across the region but not everywhere. Above all it is an urban phenomenon, characterizing many of the larger urban areas. It penetrates rural areas only when these areas are developed economically and educationally. Thus fertility decline is occurring generally in southern Africa, the Central Province of Kenya, the eastern and Volta regions of Ghana, and across southern Nigeria. Indeed, in West Africa a major regional locus of fertility decline can be discerned stretching from Abidjan to Yaoundé, including all the cities in between and much of the rural population.

In one sense this is classic demographic transition: child mortality fell, levels of urbanization rose, and income levels and those of female education increased. But this is not the whole story. Society, in a way that was difficult to perceive or even measure, was changing. Children were more likely to stay within their nuclear families, and the parents of such families, especially in the towns, were more likely to be bearing most of the cost of their upbringing. The parents, too, were more alert to the need for the children to receive adequate health care and more prolonged schooling. Just as the changes achieved momentum they were challenged by the occurrence of economic crises and the cures promoted for it after the mid-1980s. Incomes stopped rising and the cost of schooling and health treatment climbed steeply. Because the modern sector of employment henceforth grew only slowly, parents became more desperate to keep their children at school to become educated enough to grasp the opportunities that remained, and adolescent girls became more determined that pregnancy followed by a birth would not thwart their chances of finishing their schooling and getting and holding a modern-sector job. Higher incomes and education were still associated with the greatest fertility control, but that control was exercised ever more strictly, precisely because there were no more advances in these areas.

This is a situation that all the studies in this book support. The studies are of great value in that they put flesh on to the DHS's statistical proof that fertility decline is underway. They show how and why the mechanisms operate to postpone or forgo births, and their findings rarely conflict. They show how in contemporary Africa couples and governments react to the new circumstances. Most governments have lost their belief that fertility control is at odds with the "African way," although many retain sufficient fear that this idea might have some validity not to show too much enthusiasm for the necessary family planning programs.

The studies show such a high level of nonmarital sexual activity, whether among urban, middle-class adolescents in Mali or everyone in Nairobi's slums, that it is clear that adolescent girls are in great danger of pregnancy and that much of the community is threatened by HIV infection. They also show that any policy to lessen either threat that is anchored almost solely in advocating the restriction of sexual relations to within marriage, and ignores issues of sexuality and the need for a massive provision of condoms to adolescents and others, together with a realistic and sympathetic understanding of nonmarital sexual activity, is doomed to failure and could be regarded as cruel. Nonmarital sexual activity will continue because most people do not regard it as heinous or unforgivable, and because many females receive money or presents in return that meet needs ranging from the purchase of modern clothes to the prevention of family starvation.

Most of the researchers would probably agree with the findings from Ndola that there is little difference between those couples practicing contraception and those with unmet needs. In most cases there is a lack of certainty about the economic and social costs and returns from fertility. It is often chance that separates the two groups. Most would be controlling fertility if governments and the bureaucracy were more certain about the need to do so, and repeatedly expressed that message loudly, and if the family planning provision were sufficiently organized. Where these conditions are not met at all, as in the Sudan irrigation project, then even a society meeting all the other development conditions may maintain high fertility.

The first condition is a high government and elite profile in family planning. But African heads of state and their ministers rarely give such leadership and rarely say pointedly that families and nations would benefit from lower fertility. Most of them probably now believe it, and some may even be overoptimistic that a fertility decline would reverse the economic downturn, but they do not believe that identification with the issue would increase their political support. Most suffer, as do politicians elsewhere, from very short policy time horizons. The parallel with their lack of prominent leadership in combating AIDS is obvious.

The second condition is family planning programs that meet all the specific needs. African family planning clinics are becoming more efficient, but in the style of the Asian clinics catering entirely to married women. The research reported here, as well as other research reported by Caldwell and Caldwell (2001), is unanimous that the clinics are not getting any better at reaching adolescents or men with either supplies or empathy. Indeed, it is reported here that the clinics are alienating men, and thus making them hostile to allowing their wives to use modern contraception and explaining much of the unmet need. The evidence is the same as it was years ago with regard to adolescents, namely that they are most unlikely to get contraceptive help from the family planning programs. Again, the parallel with AIDS is obvious.

The way forward in sub-Saharan Africa is no mystery. The demand is for birth spacing and for short-term methods that can prevent premarital or extramarital conceptions. More than anywhere else in the world it is for hormonal methods. The only highly organized program in sub-Saharan Africa, that in South Africa, halved black African fertility in one-third of a century by meeting the demand for injectables and contraceptive pills. It did this in spite of having been set up by a hated apartheid government that could not adopt high-profile leadership and, accordingly, in the face of considerable suspicion from men (but not women) in the political resistance movement. On the whole there was no pressure (except apparently in individual factories or farms) because the government could not afford to incite opposition in what was not regarded as a core policy area.

The summary in the above paragraph is subject to some modification. The total number of suitable methods in sub-Saharan Africa could include other hormonal contraception such as Norplant. There is some evidence that neither IUDs nor female sterilization can be ruled out, although their use on any scale will almost certainly mean bringing men much more into discussions than most programs now do. There has to be a role for condoms, given the HIV/AIDS situation, but the evidence remains that their use within marriage or other unions of some permanence is likely to be small. Abortion, increasingly by doctors and illegal but not pursued by police or government, is apparently the unmeasured phenomenon that explains why some of the fertility declines have been more rapid and greater than the contraceptive prevalence rates would have predicted. Zambia has long had legal abortion under onerous conditions, and South Africa now has a liberal abortion law, but the evidence seems to be that legal abortion will not play a major role in the immediate future in promoting fertility decline. In contrast, as the number of doctors increases, illegal medical abortion may assume ever greater significance.

Nevertheless, the sub-Saharan African fertility transition still has a long way to go. With regard to the threshold characteristics for fertility decline, which we set out slightly differently in two papers (Caldwell et al. 1992; Caldwell and Caldwell 1993), some sub-Saharan African countries will not reach these levels until the middle of the present century. Only one-third of individual districts in the region as yet show any signs of decline (Tabutin and Schoumaker 2001). This is largely a matter of low levels of sociodemographic development. But a history of family planning activity also counts. At the 1965 Belgrade International Population Conference, the prediction was made that such activity would ensure that anglophone Africa took the lead in fertility decline (Caldwell 1966, pp. 164–167). Among the 13 areas of sub-Saharan Africa now leading the decline, 85 percent are anglophone and 15 percent francophone, and among a broader group of 32 with significant decline, 78 percent are anglophone, 16 percent francophone, and 6 percent Portuguese-speaking

Finally, one further observation is called for. If the greatest demand is for contraception to substitute for traditional methods of birth spacing, then, as the period of postpartum sexual abstinence shortens with modernization, and contraceptive replacement lags behind, a rise in fertility might be expected. This did happen in many societies (Romaniuk 1980). Then a fall to the original level but no further might be anticipated. This has not happened, and in many places fertility has fallen further. The basic reason is a familiarity with contraception no matter what its original purpose. It maintains the birth interval better than some of the traditional methods. It can be used to achieve an increasingly desired longer interval. By extending the final interval it can be used, even by women or couples who do not admit it to themselves, to effect birth limitation, or it can consciously be used for this purpose. Once contraception is available and widely known it can be used to prevent premarital and extramarital conceptions. Through a combination of these purposes, the sub-Saharan African fertility transition has begun in the region as a whole and in perhaps one-third of its constituent subareas.

REFERENCES

Brass, William, and Carole L. Jolly (1993). *Population Dynamics of Kenya*. Washington, DC: National Academy Press.

Caldwell, John C. (1966). Africa. In Bernard Berelson et al. (eds.). *Family Planning and Population Programs: A Review of World Developments*. Chicago: University of Chicago Press, pp. 163–181.

Caldwell, John C. (1968). *Population Growth and Family Change in Africa*. Canberra: Australian National University Press.

Caldwell, John C., and Pat Caldwell (1987). The cultural context of high fertility in sub-Saharan Africa. *Population and Development Review*, vol. 13, no. 3, pp. 409–437.

Caldwell, John C., and Pat Caldwell (1993). The South African fertility decline. *Population and Development Review*, vol. 19, no. 2, pp. 225–262.

Caldwell, John C., and Pat Caldwell (2001). Sub-Saharan family planning programs in the 20th and 21st centuries. In John C. Caldwell, James F. Phillips and Barkat-e-Khuda (eds.). *Family Planning Programs in the Twenty-first Century. Studies in Family Planning* 33(1): 76–86.

Caldwell, John C., I.O. Orubuloye, and Pat Caldwell (1992). Fertility decline in Africa: a new type of transition. *Population and Development Review*, vol. 18, no. 2, pp. 211–242.

Gueye, Mouhamadou, Sarah Castle, and Mamadou Kani Konaté (2001). Timing of first intercourse among Malian adolescents: implications for contraceptive use. *International Family Planning Perspectives*, vol. 27, no. 2, pp. 56–62, 70.

Maddison, Angus (1995). *Monitoring the World Economy, 1820–1992*. Paris: Development Centre, Organization for Economic Cooperation & Development.

Maddison, Angus (1999). Economic progress: the last half century in historical perspective. Paper presented at Academy of Social Sciences in Australia, 1999 Symposium: Facts and Fancies of Human Development, Canberra, November 8.

Mahy, Mary, and Neeru Gupta. (2001). Trends and differentials in age at first birth in sub-Saharan Africa. Paper presented at International Union for the Scientific Study of Population, 24th IUSSP General Population Conference, Salvador, Brazil, August 18–24.

Romaniuk, Anatole (1980). Increase in natural fertility during the early stages of modernization: evidence from an African case study, Zaire. *Population Studies*, vol. 34, no. 2, pp. 293–310.

Tabutin, Dominique, and Bruno Schoumaker (2001). Une analyse régionale des transitions de fécondité en Afrique sub-saharienne. Paper presented at International Union for the Scientific Study of Population, 24th IUSSP General Population Conference, Salvador, Brazil, August 18–24.

United Nations (1999). *World Population Prospects: The 1998 Revision*, vol. 1, *Comprehensive Tables*. New York.

World Bank (2001). *World Development Report 2000/2001*. New York: Oxford University Press.

Index

About the Editors and Contributors

SAMUEL AGYEI-MENSAH is Senior Lecturer, Department of Geography and Resource Development, University of Ghana. He received his Ph.D. in 1997 from the Norwegian University of Science and Technology, Trondheim, Norway. He has conducted research on a blend of issues that lie at the interface of medical geography, demography, and development studies. His most recent publications include *Fertility Decline in Developing Countries, 1960–1997: An Annotated Bibliography*, Greenwood Press (1999); "Patterns of fertility change in Ghana: a time and space perspective" (with A. Aase), *Geografiska Annaler* (1998); and "Twelve years of HIV/AIDS in Ghana: puzzles of interpretation," *Canadian Journal of African Studies* (2001). He is currently working on a manuscript on the population of Ghana. Samuel Agyei-Mensah serves on the International Advisory Board, Population, Environment Research Network of the International Union for the Scientific Study of Population (IUSSP).

JOHN B. CASTERLINE is Senior Research Associate, Policy Research Division, Population Council, New York, USA. He received his Ph.D. in 1980 from the University of Michigan. Most of his research career has been devoted to investigation of reproductive behavior, in particular the determinants and consequences of fertility transition. Recent publications include "Unmet need for family planning in developing countries and implications for population policy" (with S. Sinding), *Population and Development Review* (2000); *Global Fertility Transition* (coedited with Rodolfo Bulatao), supplement to *Population and Development Review* (2001); and *Diffusion Processes and Fertility Transition,* National Academy Press (2001). He is currently involved in research on demographic transition in the Arab region, social diffusion and reproductive behavior in West Africa, and unintended fertility in Pakistan. He has served on the Board of Directors of the Population Association of America, the Committee on the Comparative Analysis of Fertility of the IUSSP, and the Committee on Population of the National Academy of Sciences. He is currently a member of the Panel on Social Science and Operations Research in Reproductive Health, the World Health Organization.

ASBJORN AASE is Professor of Geography, Norwegian University of Science and Technology, Trondheim, Norway.

DOMINIC K. AGYEMAN is Professor of Sociology, University of Cape Coast, Cape Coast, Ghana.

KOFI AWUSABO-ASARE is Associate Professor of Geography, University of Cape Coast, Ghana.

BETEMARIAM BERHANU is Assistant Vice-President, Acquisition Credit Policy, Citibank, USA.

ANN E. BIDDLECOM is Research Investigator, Institute for Social Research, University of Michigan, USA.

JOHN C. CALDWELL is Emeritus Professor of Demography, Australian National University, Canberra, Australia.

PAT CALDWELL is Visitor, Health Transition Center, Australian National University, Canberra, Australia.

SARAH CASTLE is Lecturer, Centre for Population Studies, London School of Hygiene and Tropical Medicine, University of London, UK.

F. NII-AMOO DODOO is Professor and Chair, Afro-American Studies Program, and Center on Population, Gender and Social Inequality, University of Maryland, USA.

DENNIS P. HOGAN is Robert E. Turner Distinguished Professor of Population Studies and Professor of Sociology, Brown University, USA.

EZEKIEL KALIPENI is Associate Professor of Geography, University of Illinois, Urbana-Champaign, USA.

FREDERICK A.D. KAONA is Director, Mwengu Social and Health Research Centre, Ndola, Zambia.

MAMADOU KANI KONATE is Programme Officer, Gender, Family and Development Programme, Centre d'Etudes et de Recherche sur la Population pour le Developpement (CERPOD), Bamako, Mali.

EL-RAYAH A. OSMAN is Associate Professor of Sociology, Department of Psychology and Sociology, South Carolina State University, USA.

MELISSA SLOAN is Doctoral Student, Department of Sociology, Vanderbilt University, USA.

ELIYA MSIYAPHAZI ZULU is Senior Research Scientist, African Population and Health Research Center, Nairobi, Kenya.

www.ingramcontent.com/pod-product-compliance
Ingram Content Group UK Ltd.
Pitfield, Milton Keynes, MK11 3LW, UK
UKHW020815290926
15470UKWH00003B/1162

9 780313 319082